Verna Rickard, BSW, LS

The Learning About Myself (LAMS) Program for At-Risk Parents
Learning from the Past— Changing the Future

Pre-publication REVIEWS, COMMENTARIES, EVALUATIONS . . .

"This is an excellent program. The LAMS materials are designed to meet the clients where they are. I found the information to be extremely practical, down-to-earth, and applicable to daily living. The author makes every attempt to address the clients' needs realistically.

The LAMS program provides the client with a firm foundation of information on which to build. I particularly appreciated Ms. Rickard's emphasis on individual choice and the importance of positive attitudes. This program should be a part of the resource materials of every mental health professional who works with at-risk parents."

Terry King, PhD
*Clinical Psychologist,
Federal Bureau of Prisons,
Catlettsburg, KY*

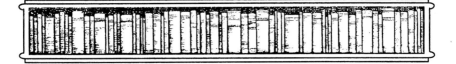

More pre-publication
REVIEWS, COMMENTARIES, EVALUATIONS . . .

"**F**or those in the child welfare field who have lost hope that public child welfare agencies can truly respond to the needs of parents who abuse and neglect their children, Verna Rickard's *LAMS Program for At-Risk Parents* proves otherwise. Rickard has developed a structured, fifteen-session group intervention for parents whose isolation, lack of education, and minimal social skills place them at high risk for maltreating their children. The LAMS curriculum was honed over a seven-year period of testing with just such parents.

The LAMS Program is more than just another parent training program, most of which have proven ineffective in changing abusive or neglectful parenting behavior. Rickard draws on recent empirical studies of abusive and neglectful parents to design a curriculum that addresses the true complexity of maltreating parents' lives. Studies show that maltreating parents suffer from low self-esteem, have limited problem-solving skills, have attenuated social networks, and have, themselves, frequently been physically and sexually abused. Through the LAMS Program, parents are helped to develop a better understanding and acceptance of themselves, to improve their relationships to the world around them, and to acquire knowledge and skills for better functioning in everyday life. This is done through a structured series of group activities specifically designed with the educational and cognitive limitations experienced by many maltreating parents in mind. Best of all, not only is the LAMS Program designed to be educational and build skills for future use, it is also FUN! Most parents who begin the program finish it and many come back for more—a sharp contrast to the high dropout rates of most parenting programs, even those where parents are mandated to attend.

A close look at the *LAMS Program for At-Risk Parents* is highly recommended for all those working in the child welfare field who truly want to make a difference in the lives of maltreating parents and their children."

Martha Morrison Dore, PhD
Associate Professor of Social Work,
Columbia University
School of Social Work

The Learning About Myself (LAMS) Program for At-Risk Parents

Learning from the Past— Changing the Future

THE HAWORTH MALTREATMENT & TRAUMA PRESS
Robert A. Geffner, PhD
Editor

The Learning About Myself (LAMS) Program for At-Risk Parents
Learning from the Past— Changing the Future

Verna Rickard, BSW, LSW

HMTP

The Haworth Maltreatment and Trauma Press
An Imprint of The Haworth Press, Inc.

Published by

The Haworth Maltreatment and Trauma Press, an imprint of The Haworth Press, Inc., 10 Alice Street, Binghamton, NY 13904-1580

Cover design by Monica L. Seifert.

Library of Congress Cataloging-in-Publication Data

Rickard, Verna.
　　The learning about myself (LAMS) program for at-risk parents : learning from the past— changing the future / Verna Rickard.
　　　　p.　cm.
　　Includes bibliographical references and index.
　　ISBN 0-7890-0474-7 (alk. paper).
　　1. Parenting—Study and teaching. 2. Self-actualization (Psychology). I. Title.
HQ755.7.R53 1998
158.1′085—dc21　　　　　　　　　　　　　　　　　　　　　　　　　97-45068
　　　　　　　　　　　　　　　　　　　　　　　　　　　　　　　　CIP

CONTENTS

ABOUT THE AUTHOR

Verna Rickard, BSW, LSW, is a Child Protective Service Specialist IV for the Texas Department of Protective and Regulatory Services, an organization she has worked for since 1979. Her many years of casework in intensive home-based services to high-risk abusive and neglectful families led to the development of the Learning About Myself (LAMs) program in 1990. Since then she has taught the LAMs program weekly. She has presented the program and its concepts to the Regional Child Welfare board, at the Governor's Conferences on the Prevention of Child Abuse in Austin, Texas, in 1995 and 1996; at the National Association for Family Based Services Conferences in Texas and Minnesota in 1996 and 1997; and at a homeless shelter for the Fort Worth Independent School District.

If your agency has questions or would like in-person assistance in setting up or training facilitators for the LAMS program, contact Verna Rickard in Fort Worth, Texas, by phone at (817) 246-9215.

CONTRIBUTOR

Marianne Berry, PhD, ACSW, is an Associate Professor of Social Work at the University of Texas at Arlington. She is a founder of the UTA Center for Child Welfare. She received her doctorate in social welfare from the University of California, Berkeley, and her master's degree in social service administration from the University of Chicago. She is the author or co-author of more than forty refereed journal articles and book chapters on a variety of child welfare issues. She has authored or co-authored three books: a book on older child adoptions, *Adoption and Disruption* (Aldine de Gruyter), and two on intensive family preservation services, *Keeping Families Together* (Garland Publishing), and *The Family at Risk: Issues and Trends in Family Preservation Services* (The University of South Carolina Press). She is on the editorial board of *Children and Youth Services Review, Family Preservation Journal,* and *Child and Family Social Work.* She is a Research Fellow of the American Association of University Women. She received the Frank Breul Memorial Prize from the *Social Service Review* for outstanding scholarship in child welfare.

Acknowledgments

I would like to thank my longtime supervisor, Jere Fenton, and my co-workers in Unit 31 for their constant encouragement and support in getting LAMS from concept to publication. LAMS has been field-tested for over five years by our Family Preservation Unit as part of its ongoing client services. Caseworker Anna Bowen was my first co-facilitator, and presently, Dottie Dixon fills that role. Sarah Jameson attended all the sessions as part of her field placement and also helped out in many ways. Countless others, including group members, students, and volunteers, have assisted over the years of development. Marianne Berry, an Associate Professor of Social Work at the University of Texas at Arlington, has done past research on the content and effectiveness of the LAMS program and is presently conducting another research study with doctoral student Scottye Cash.

Dottie Dixon and Sarah Jameson reviewed the manuscript to ensure that the instructions were simple and comprehensive.

Thank you also to my family, who had to live with my unavailability while I was typing the many modifications and revisions of the original LAMS program.

PART ONE:
PROGRAM

Chapter 1

What Is LAMS?

LAMS is a fifteen-week basic, hands-on, group curriculum that helps change participants' lives from hopeless and helpless to confident and self-assured. It helps explain how past experiences affect the present, teaches basic skills, and creates observable changes in appearance, confidence, and self-image. Participants learn to cope with life rather than being overwhelmed by problems.

Positive affirmations, games, and other activities are selected to support the topic for each week. Lecture, group discussion, and role-plays are used to explain how to make better decisions, set goals, and live life by "choice," not by "chance." This is an open-ended curriculum. If the series is completed in any order, the benefits should remain the same.

The language is simple to understand, and the program is easily adaptable to all ages and both sexes. It can be used as an introduction to individual counseling or as the primary treatment.

The leader of this course does not need to be a therapist, only someone with a basic knowledge of social work, psychological concepts, or life skills.

SUPPORTING RESEARCH

Programs to prevent or reduce the abuse and neglect of children have proliferated over the past several decades, as public awareness of child abuse and its long-term effects has grown. Educational and support groups, such as Learning About Myself, are effective means to teach and support parents in the use of positive coping strategies and thought patterns that can result in better parenting and family functioning.

Raising happy children requires happy parents. Families with abused or neglected children are often termed multiproblem families or families out of control (Garbarino, 1977). There is a wealth of empirical research on the correlates of child mistreatment. Child abuse has been associated with many parenting stressors such as large amounts of time spent between parent and child (Johnson and L'Esperance, 1984), low levels of parenting skills (Johnson and L'Esperance, 1984), illness of the mother (Sherrod et al., 1984), young age of the mother (Young and Gately, 1988), and presence of multiple children in the home (Johnson and L'Esperance, 1984). Child characteristics that have been associated with abuse and neglect include child illness or abnormalities (Sherrod et al., 1984), difficult child temperament (Sherrod et al., 1984), and provocative or difficult child behavior (Paulson et al., 1975).

Parents who abuse or neglect their children often have histories of deprivation, mental illness, and low self-esteem (Gaines et al., 1978; Garbarino, 1976; Paulson et al., 1975; Shapiro, 1980), and are often, but not always, from a lower socioeconomic group (Garbarino, 1976; Shapiro, 1980). They are also likely to suffer marital difficulties, unemployment, unwanted pregnancy and crowded living conditions (Parke and Collmer, 1975).

Clearly, the stressors facing families who abuse or neglect their children are many. Research in child abuse and neglect indicates that maltreating parents are likely to have few or impotent resources with which to cope (Johnson and L'Esperance, 1984; McClelland, 1973), particularly, little social support (Paulson et al., 1975; Wein-

"Supporting Research" is contributed by Marianne Berry, PhD, ACSW, an Associate Professor of Social Work at the University of Texas at Arlington, specializing in child welfare policy and programs.

traub and Wolf, 1983). They are isolated from social networks and other sources of modeling and support (Polansky and Gaudin, 1983). This isolation and lack of resources, financial and social, contributes to unhappy mothers and fathers who are easily stressed and undone by the demands of children.

Given that parenting is often the primary responsibility of mothers (whether in single- or dual-parent households), it is not surprising that child abuse is one area of violence where women are perpetrators in equal proportions to men (Breines and Gordon, 1983; Young and Gately, 1988). Research has found that mothers in abusive families and socially isolated families have fewer than average positive exchanges within the family and greater than average negative exchanges (Patterson, 1982). In other words, mothers often bear the brunt of the stress and isolation of families and are the recipients of patterns of aggression within the family. These patterns, over time, provide a stressful and demanding family environment and decrease the number of positive interactions and resources for mothers (Patterson, 1980).

Wahler and Dumas (1984) have identified abuse as occurring in families with insular mothers. Insularity is defined as "a specific pattern of social contacts within the community that are characterized by a high level of negatively perceived coercive interchanges with relatives and/or helping agency representatives and by a low level of positively perceived supportive interchanges with friends" (Wahler and Dumas, 1984, p. 387). Those children with insular mothers are at risk of abuse because these mothers have limited opportunities to diffuse stress and also have few models of positive interaction. Therefore, social and educational support groups for these mothers can be extremely effective in helping to diffuse the stress and in helping to manage day-to-day stress without abusing their children.

Research on the prevention of therapy for child maltreatment is not as plentiful as that on correlates of abuse or the placement of children in foster homes. This reflects an emphasis in research and mental health services on the diagnosis of problems rather than the solving of problems. Nevertheless, evaluations of child abuse prevention and treatment programs to date have identified several components and frameworks that are correlated with program effectiveness.

Berry (1988) conducted a review of all evaluation research on parent-training programs in child welfare services and found that programs to prevent child abuse are much more likely to be didactic than interactive. However, the interactive programs (such as the Learning About Myself groups outlined in this manuscript) were found to be more effective than didactic programs in demonstrating behavior changes in the parents and in producing effects that were still evident at follow-up visits. These interactive and behavioral programs (Forehand and McMahon, 1981; Patterson, Chamberlain, and Reid, 1982) train parents in increasing social rewards to children, giving clear commands, and rewarding compliance.

Dumas (1986) and others (Griest and Forehand, 1982; Lovell, Reid, and Richey, 1992) have found that socioeconomic stressors and a lack of social support inhibit short-term gains during parent training and minimize the longevity of the effects. In their article, "How can I get any parent training done with all those other problems going on?", Griest and Forehand (1982) reported that child behavior problems were associated with parent adjustment problems, marital problems, and extrafamilial problems and that these problems often interfere with the maintenance of parent-training effects. Similarly, Lovell, Reid, and Richey (1992) found, in their parent-training group for abusive parents, that "it was not uncommon for parent group members unwittingly to respond to each other with embarrassing and/or inappropriate comments. They appeared genuinely surprised to learn that their remarks were offensive or hurtful to others . . . In general, mothers appeared unable to give and receive social support" (p. 96).

Both Forehand and colleagues (Forehand and McMahon, 1981; Griest and Forehand, 1982) and Patterson and colleagues (Patterson, 1982; Patterson, Chamberlain, and Reid, 1982) now emphasize that groups and training to prevent and reduce child abuse must be expanded to include what they call a "parent-enhancement" component. A parent-enhancement component focuses on the perceptions and expectations of the parent about the child's behavior, the parent's mood and psychological adjustment, spouse-partner communication, problem solving, and the parent's interactions outside the family. In other words, training must focus on the parent as a person, not just as a parent, and must address decision making, positive self-esteem, making good choices, and considering consequences, and much more, as presented in the Learning About Myself groups.

In their seminal review of child abuse prevention programs, Cohn and Daro (1987) surmise that, " . . . successful intervention with maltreating families requires a comprehensive package which addresses both the interpersonal and concrete needs of all family members" (p. 437). Raising happy children requires happy parents, and Learning About Myself is a group experience that addresses the whole person, not just parenting skills. This comprehensiveness is grounded in and supported by research in child abuse prevention.

HISTORY OF THE PROGRAM

Effective programs that prevent or reduce the risk of abuse and neglect of children are becoming more and more important as the number of such cases has climbed in recent years. The past emphasis of research and mental health services has been more on diagnosing problems than on solving them. Griest and Forehand (1982) reported that child behavior problems went hand in hand with his or her parent's adjustment problems, marital problems, and extrafamilial problems. They went on to say that such problems often interfere with the parent's ability to parent his or her children well. LAMS is a program that deals with the parent's past before it affects the child's future.

The LAMS program originated in the Intensive Family Preservation Unit, part of the Texas Department of Protective and Regulatory Services/Child Protective Services, in Fort Worth, Texas. It was developed to help women involved with Child Protective Services learn to understand and take control of their lives.

Many of these women dropped out of school in early high school years, usually because of pregnancy, leaving them poorly equipped for adulthood. Most were on some type of public assistance and remained single parents. A few were living with or married to their children's fathers. Fewer still were working or had adequate incomes to support their families. They felt hopeless, helpless, and depressed—adults still functioning as children. They wanted to be good parents but were unable to give their children the love and attention they needed because they never received it themselves. They were survivors who had managed to stay afloat in rowboats but who needed to be taught to build ships.

These women, typical Family Preservation clients, had not shown improvement when referred to out-of-agency contracted groups. They complained that everything said there was "over their heads." Education of some type was imperative if they were to make the necessary changes in their lives. After discussion, it was determined that case-workers *themselves* were the ones with the most experience with clients' families and the ones most aware of their special needs. If outside agencies could not provide what was needed, then in-agency caseworkers would have to find a way to do so.

Verna Rickard, with a social work degree and over thirteen years experience, had a longtime interest in working with neglectful and unmotivated mothers so she began research to discover what was needed to help those women understand and take control of their lives. Many such clients felt life just "happened" to them, and there was nothing they could do to change their situations.

Research of current literature and consultations with therapists and group leaders in the area showed that little had been done to meet the needs of such women. There were groups that treated individual facets of their problems but nothing that combined everything in one course. The LAMS program was developed to include what researchers felt was valuable, what group leaders thought was missing in what they were teaching, and what caseworkers observed to be clients' needs.

A study by Garbarino (1977) pointed out that multiproblem families have more children who are abused and neglected. Young and Gately (1988) said young mothers, especially those with multiple children, tended to be associated with difficult children, child abnormalities, and ultimately, child abuse and neglect. Other studies done in the 1970s (Paulson et al., 1975; Gaines et al., 1978; Garbarino, 1976) showed that parental histories of deprivation, mental illness, and low self-esteem contributed to abuse and neglect. It was concluded that the problems of the *parents* had to be addressed before those of their children—and it had to be done in language easily understood by women with low educational levels. It also had to be done in a manner that would keep group members coming back. Despite the caveat that families served by public child welfare agencies are poor candidates for group participation and attendance (Polansky, Ammons, and Gaudin, 1985; Polansky et al., 1981), our LAMS group has had a very good attendance and participation rate over several years.

Out-of-agency therapists were asked what they thought needed to be included in classes in order to reach our clients and what concepts they wished were a part of their curriculum. Their suggestions included simplifying the language, presenting basic concepts at an easily understandable level, and teaching more practical skills. All of their ideas were added to what had been learned from research and what caseworkers knew about the Child Protective Services client base. The LAMS program was the result.

Development began in the summer of 1990, and the program was first taught in October of that year. Originally, LAMS was taught only to mothers, but several fathers wanted to attend and were included. As of February 1997, more than 400 participants have attended at least one and usually several of the classes. Over 100 have graduated, including several men.

Many clients cannot finish the program because their cases have been closed, or they go to work or move. Others have had to leave because of illness or family problems. Some attend once or twice and never return, but if they attend several times, they usually complete the program.

Therapists have commented that when individual counseling follows LAMS group, the participants recognize basic principles and say, "Oh, I know about that—we learned it in LAMS."

Post-group evaluations by participants and caseworkers show that group members have made changes in their lives because of things they learned in LAMS. One hundred percent of the clients, for whom full information was available (see appendix for 1997 study by Marianne Berry, PhD), said they believed that individuals who feel helpless can learn to be more powerful, and 90 percent said they now feel they have choices and that life no longer just "happens" to them. Over 25 percent of the group members had tried something they used to be afraid of while attending the LAMS group. All said they had increased their social supports, with an average of five new friends per client. This is significant because most were very isolated when they began attending.

Clients felt that learning to make choices was the most important skill they gained from attending the LAMS program (90 percent); ranked next in importance was experiencing warm relationships in the group (79 percent). They also felt they learned to be more assertive and to identify and accept feelings.

Caseworkers also felt that Learning About Myself was an effective experience for their clients (see appendix). Improvements in clients' self-esteem were noted in 89 percent, in their children's appearance, 53 percent, and greater independence in 44 percent. Almost all caseworkers felt attendance at LAMS would contribute to earlier closure of their clients' Child Protective Services cases.

Historical Problems

Development of the LAMS program has not been without problems. The largest ones have been transportation, child care, and money for supplies. All three are equally necessary to the success of the group. Most of our families have little money; few have cars, and the mass-transit system covers only parts of this county. Many are isolated so have no friends or relatives to provide child care when necessary. Certain activities and providing refreshments made a funding source necessary.

Transportation was at first provided by caseworkers, case aides, and clients who had enough money for bus fare or access to a car. Occasionally, several women in the same area would ride with the one who had a car. Churches and other organizations with vans or buses were contacted, unsuccessfully. Lack of funding prohibited contracting with taxi companies, as some local private agencies do. Later, our agency had a contract with a homemaker service provider that included transporting our families, but that was short-lived. Currently, all of the transportation is provided by agency workers or the clients themselves, though sometimes bus tokens can be provided by our agency.

At first, mothers brought their children with them to LAMS, and a play area was set up away from the meeting space with supervision by a co-worker. This did not work well, as it was too distracting. Later, the meeting location was changed, and the large room could be divided by a folding partition. Shortly after that, homemakers watched the children after bringing the families to the group. Now a different contracted homemaker agency provides one child care attendant weekly, and our case aide assists. If there are several children, other unit members help out.

Funding was initially the responsibility of the LAMS facilitator, and only snacks and drinks were provided. Any projects had to be personally funded or were donated. Second-year expenses were covered by a grant from a local department store. Expenses are now covered in the county's Child Welfare Board budget, which enables a much broader scope of activities. A full meal is provided weekly, craft and holiday projects arc included, and the Pretty Prize, a weekly door prize of beauty products, can be given. Donations of goods and supplies still augment budgeted items.

Your agency may have no problems in any of these areas, but these comments were included to show how seemingly insurmountable problems can be overcome and how the LAMS program can be adapted to various situations.

GOALS OF THE LAMS PROGRAM

Educational and support groups such as LAMS are effective in teaching parents positive coping skills and thought patterns that result in healthier families. Research by Polansky and Gaudin (1983) determined that parents isolated from social support systems were easily stressed and were less able to withstand the demands of their children. These support systems are the source of most skills learned by parents. At-risk parents seldom have family or friends to advise them and may never learn parenting, housekeeping, or social skills.

The first goal of LAMS is to teach basic skills for dealing with life. Women, or men, who do not feel they *have* choices, are unable to *make* choices. LAMS teaches needed skills to help participants recognize when decisions have to be made and how to make them wisely. It helps them understand that insults they heard as children were not necessarily true, and they may be more competent than they realize. It helps them set goals for themselves and learn how planning can help them reach those goals. Most of all, it helps them realize that they are persons different from everyone else, with their own skills, desires, and capabilities—persons whose lives are just beginning.

The next goal of LAMS is to help these same women, or men, learn to get along better with others—in their family relationships, with friends, and in the community. Some may need to change their attitude, possibly be less passive or aggressive. Interactions in the group are helpful to members who in the past have found it hard to make friends or who may be estranged from their families.

Third, some participants need help with practical things, such as getting more education, job training, or getting a job to increase their income to provide better care for their family. The goal of LAMS is to provide information in these areas and instill in clients the confidence that they need to accomplish their goals.

Finances, sensible shopping, and nutrition are often problematic areas for these women. Many of them had poor examples at home and did not attend school long enough to learn much about such subjects. LAMS provides information on basic budgeting, comparative shopping, and on foods that provide proper nutrition for their families.

Since low self-esteem and depression often cause our clients to be apathetic about their appearance, instruction is provided on good grooming, makeup, clothing, and colors that help them look their best. Their appearance almost always improves, sometimes dramatically, from their first class and throughout the program.

All through the LAMS program affirmations are used that help change "self-talk" from negative to positive. Activities are geared toward success for everyone, whatever their capacity. They learn that they deserve time for themselves and that they have feelings and desires which can be expressed. They also learn that they do *not* have to be victims of physical abuse, and they do not *deserve* to be punished, whatever their background.

The final goal is to address the *whole* person, not just the *parent-*person. After completion of the LAMS program, participants will be able to understand and take control of their lives and realize that they can change their lives for the better.

Preliminary research on the Learning About Myself program has been completed by Marianne Berry, PhD, from the University of Texas at Arlington. Her findings are listed in the appendix. Findings show that the goals are being met and that the LAMS program is an effective tool in changing the lives of those who participate.

WHO CAN BENEFIT?

LAMS program benefits can be documented by recent research in the welfare field. Research done by Berry (1988) reviewed parent-training programs in child welfare agencies. Dr. Berry did additional research in 1996/1997 (see appendix). This confirmed that both clients and caseworkers saw positive changes in clients' lives after they completed the LAMS program.

The LAMS program can be adapted for use with many types of clients. The client base of Child Protective Services is extremely varied. The sole common denominator is that all are parents, though the number and age of their children is different in most cases. The youngest mother to attend LAMS was fourteen, and the oldest client was a great-grandmother of the children involved. One seventeen-year-old client was already the mother of five children, and many others have been close to that record.

Many of the persons who attended LAMS had problems with reading or comprehension, and most had dropped out of school before tenth grade. They had great difficulty understanding out-of-agency presentations of information on parenting or self-improvement so often did not continue to attend.

Consequently, the language of the LAMS program is intentionally kept very simple; however, it does not "talk down" to anyone and can be used on any educational level. Terms such as "passive," "assertive," and "aggressive" have been reduced to a basic level to increase understanding. In addition, demonstrations by the leaders and role-plays by group participants enable everyone to learn the real "meaning" of the concepts. LAMS has been successfully completed by several persons who were unable to read and write and by many others with very limited skills. All written material is read aloud, and any questions are read one at a time and completed by the group as a whole. If someone in the group seems to be having problems with an activity, the person next to them is asked to help, or one of the leaders does so.

Abusive parents often have histories of mental illness. Several persons who are mentally challenged have completed the LAMS program. Mental problems encompass both retardation and mental illness. One such woman was asked to leave the program due to her argumentative and aggressive behavior, but she wanted to come back. She was allowed to do so after promising to do better and went through the program three times because she enjoyed coming. She eventually learned the concepts and was able to put them into practice. Several other persons who were mentally challenged did very well even though they were unable to read or write. They learned valuable skills and also enjoyed the social aspects of the group.

LAMS seems to work exceptionally well with women who are in drug rehabilitation programs. Some of the most successful graduates, those who made the most changes in their lives, have been in such programs. Possibly, they are more motivated to put what they learn into practice because they realize they have had unmanageable problems in the past and want to learn new, effective ways of dealing with them.

A high percentage of Intensive Family Preservation clients are single parents; some are divorced, but most were never married to their children's fathers. Some were in abusive relationships, which they chose to leave; others were abandoned by the men in their lives. LAMS is effective in teaching them ways to live better lives, whether they remain single or not. Many of these women are quite bitter about all men—through LAMS, they learn to accept themselves and realize they cannot change others. They also learn how their childhood and past experiences affect their present functioning.

Parke and Collmer (1975) reported that parents with unwanted pregnancies are more likely to be abusive to those children. The LAMS program has been very effective with such women. Several young, pregnant mothers have gone through the LAMS program and learned that their lives are not over; they are just beginning. In LAMS they are taught to make better decisions and set goals for themselves. Those goals may include returning to school or entering job-training programs. Some mothers have decided to put their children up for adoption because they felt it was the best thing for all concerned; others have gained self-confidence and decided they could keep their children and make better lives for their families. They gained both personal and practical skills and found that *they* could take control of their lives.

The LAMS program was taught for several months in a homeless shelter but was discontinued because of personnel changes there.

Several of the long-term residents participated in sessions and seemed to benefit, as many of them had no idea of how to function outside of that protected setting. Many of them were well-educated but were in the shelter due to job problems, past alcohol or drug abuse, or mental conditions.

Since LAMS addresses the whole person, not just his or her parenting skills, it could be of help to prisoners prior to release, as a transition to a better life. Community counseling agencies could teach the program to at-risk parents or use it as a treatment group for parents who have already had problems. Lottie Haswell, a Presbyterian missionary to Brazil, learned of the program and said that it could even be used with the women at her outpost. *Anyone* who feels that life just "happens" to them can benefit by completing the LAMS program.

MODIFICATIONS

The LAMS program can easily be modified to fit various groups. It presently is used in both a fifteen-week and twelve-week format. To condense the program into twelve weeks, nutrition information is shortened to one week and the My Goals and Celebration weeks are combined.

Other modifications in length can easily be made by eliminating some subjects, adding others, and rearranging topics. Each week stands alone so changing the order is not disruptive. If a desired speaker is not available on a certain week, another topic can be moved to fill that time and the speaker rescheduled. Several general areas are covered. The combination makes the program different and successful, but special needs may require some changes in content.

LAMS was originally developed for women, and some small changes need to be made to accomodate mixed groups or men. In mixed groups, both male and female Pretty Prize bags need to be available so the appropriate one can be awarded to the winner of the drawing. Some crafts also need to be adapted for male participants. Men have made keyrings while the women were making hair bows, for example. Appearance week needs to concentrate on male appearance, colors, and general good grooming, as well as on makeup and hairstyles for women. Health week can easily be expanded to cover men's health issues. Many men have little understanding of women's anatomy, health, or reproduction and can benefit from much of the same information. Depending on the audience, topics can be varied. Sexually transmitted diseases, use of condoms, safe-sex issues, drug use and abuse, pregnancy, and alcoholism can all be covered. Speakers on any topic can be brought in, or it can be a more general presentation on exercise, wellness, high-blood pressure, heart disease, and necessary preventive tests. There are videos on almost any medical subject, if the equipment is available for use. Handouts add to the effectiveness of the information presented and are available from insurance companies, the American Red Cross, mental health agencies, the American Cancer Society, and other sources. Condoms can be distributed if safe-sex is an issue that needs to be addressed.

Men, as well as women, can benefit from information on budgeting, shopping, and proper nutrition. Supermarket flyers help participants compare prices and learn to plan meals around specials. Nutrition issues may depend on the clients attending; young mothers would need to know how to feed their children properly, while men would benefit from information on selecting, storing, and preparing foods. Everyone needs to know the basic food groups and what constitutes a healthy diet.

Extra emphasis on job training or education would be valuable to young persons, along with attitudes and goals for the future. Substance-abuse clients might need added information on health, choosing friends, their relationships, making decisions, and setting goals. Mental health clients possibly would need emphasis on making choices, health, appearance, and how past family experiences impact their present life.

The LAMS program is basic. Handouts, cartoons, local news articles, books, music, different games, or whatever you choose can be added to make the program fit your needs.

PART TWO: CONTENT

Chapter 2

How Do I Run the LAMS Program?

LAMS is a simple program that can be led by one person if necessary but is better led by two. With two, one can write on the board, pass out papers, or circulate around the room to help participants who are having problems. There is no necessity for the leaders to be therapists; anyone with a general understanding of basic social work or psychological principles and some life experience can be an effective facilitator.

LAMS can meet in any room large enough for your group. A chalkboard or large pad of drawing paper is needed for the group leader. Participants need writing instruments and sometimes art supplies. Chairs can be in a circle without tables, but at least one table should be available for projects that require writing, cutting, pasting, or assembly. Participants seem to prefer sitting at tables, especially if they are set up in a square or oblong so discussion is easier. Group facilitators sit at a table across the end. On weeks when crafts or other projects are part of the program, a space is left in the middle between the tables so the leaders can more easily give assistance. LAMS could be adapted to almost any setting and could even be held outdoors if basic equipment is available.

Each session of the LAMS curriculum is designed to last two and one-half hours, with a break during the middle half-hour for a meal or refreshments. The leader(s) should be in the room shortly before the session begins to get everyone settled, give instructions on how to register, and be sure everyone feels comfortable. Some method of sign-in should be used in order to track who is coming and how many weeks he or she has attended.

Some participants may never before have been part of such a group, and they may not be coming because they want to attend but because someone told them they had to. They may be defensive, timid, or argumentative, and have no idea of what to expect. Their only common bond is parenthood, and their children may live with them, with relatives, or even in foster care.

The first time they attend, new LAMS members should be given a pencil and the Pre-LAMS Questionnaire to be filled out and turned in after the meeting. This form is included as part of this chapter. The Pre-LAMS questions reveal the participants' feelings about their past, present, and future. Surprisingly, the answer given most often to the first question, "What did you never have as a child that you wanted?", is "love" or "attention." This reflects the research of Gaines and colleagues (1978), Garbarino (1976), and Shapiro (1980); parents who abuse or neglect their children have histories of deprivation and low self-esteem. The anticipated answer when this question was originally written was some *concrete object*, not an intangible such as love. The answers to the Pre-LAMS questions often reveal more about new group members than could be learned in innumerable conversations. (see Dr. Berry's 1997 study in the appendix for an analysis of the answers.)

Each new LAMS group member also receives a copy of *The LAMS Handbook for Group Participants*. The workbook, which accompanies the program, contains a week-by-week overview of the topic, the Affirmation for the week, and additional readings. It can be collected at the end of each session or taken home and brought back by the participants each week. If the handbooks are turned in weekly, there is not the "I forgot to bring it back" problem, but participants have no opportunity to read ahead or review what they learned in past sessions. If participants are allowed to take the workbooks home each week, there should be extra copies available to use during the group session in case they forget their own. At the end of the LAMS course, the workbooks should be given to the participants, who have hopefully added notes of their own to what is printed. The workbooks sometimes become dog-eared from use. One mother said she and her eight-year-old daughter often read from it between sessions.

After everyone is seated, introduce yourself and your co-leader, if there is one. Explain that this is a group, not a class, and that everyone will have a chance to discuss the topics presented. If there are new members in the group, have everyone introduce themselves, possibly giving a little personal history. Be sure all members wear name tags with at least their first names written large enough to be seen by the leaders, as well as other group members. Leaders should also wear name tags.

Next, explain any housekeeping matters, such as the location of bathrooms and water fountains, when break times will be, and where or whether smoking is allowed. Any other announcements should be made at that time also, such as cancellation of the next week's class due to a holiday and so forth. Ask if anyone has questions.

Activities can be divided between the leaders as desired, and they can sit or stand, whichever is the most comfortable for them. They may want to alternate or even walk around informally. If there are new members, or if this is your first meeting, one of the facilitators should explain the content and goals of the LAMS program. Since this is an open-ended program, each week stands alone, with a mixture of active, practical, and theoretical topics. If all fifteen weeks are completed, participants should have the information needed to change their lives for the better, but *they* will have to supply the motivation to do so. Research by Berry (1988) found that interactive programs such as LAMS were more effective than didactic programs in producing long-lasting behavior changes.

Ask that all group members turn to the Affirmation for the week being presented and give the page number. The Affirmation is read in unison and emphasizes positives. It is intended to get participants to change their thinking patterns from past negatives associated with a lack of self-esteem. The reason for reading the Affirmation aloud is to be sure that everyone hears it even if they have difficulty reading or cannot read at all. LAMS is very effective with such persons, and one of the reasons for its creation was that many Child Protective Services clients in counseling groups could not understand what was being presented by contracted agencies.

Posters that emphasize themes such as, "You can do it" and "It is better to try and fail than never to try" are often used in conjunction with the curriculum. They can be purchased in educational supply stores, as well as many other locations.

If there are additonal readings for the week, one of the leaders should read them aloud. Most are included in the handbooks, and participants can follow along. Be sure there is an opportunity for discussion and comment afterward.

A game follows the readings on most weeks. The instructions for the game are included in the general directions for the week in the leader's manual. Games are not included in the participant handbooks so will need to be thoroughly explained, and sometimes demonstrated, by the leaders. These games are planned as a part of the weekly theme and often illustrate key points that will be covered in the lesson. Many times the connection is not recognized by the group members until later in the session, when the leader may want to point out the connection. The games included in the program are survivors of five years of testing for effectiveness.

Some of the games afford opportunities for discussion of group viewpoints and how past events impact their present behavior. Group members sometimes make embarrassing or inappropriate comments that may be offensive or hurtful to others. Allowing each member of the group to answer questions helps members understand the consequences of such replies, and their peers often immediately correct or comment on such responses.

Halfway through the allotted group period there should be a thirty-minute break that includes time to share a meal. Providing food, especially a full meal, is important in building group rapport. One-dish meals can be prepared if a full kitchen is not available. Simple snacks could replace the meal if there are budgetary restrictions. The thirty-minute break enables participants to get to know each other. If child care is provided, older children can join their parents at mealtime, or they can eat in the nursery. Group interactions are valuable, as many participants have little experience getting along with others and seldom realize other people experience many of the same problems.

Depending on how long the previous activities take, the main theme for the week is presented after the break. Occasionally, if things go rapidly, you may start before the break and then continue on afterward. A complete explanation of each week's theme and how to teach it is included in the leader's guide. There is a brief overview of each lesson in the member's handbook, sometimes in greater detail, as for the shopping week and the coverage of passive, assertive, and aggressive behaviors. The *Handbook* should be used as a resource for group members during the weeks they attend and as a help to them in reviewing what they learned after they complete the LAMS course. Forehand and McMahon (1981) and Patterson and colleagues (1982) emphasized that "parent-enhancement" components that include problem solving, decision making, making good choices, and positive self-esteem are important parts of any parent-training program. These skills are all included in the curriculum of the LAMS program.

At the end of each session, evaluation forms are distributed, along with pencils if needed. A copy of this form is included as part of this chapter. The present form has been changed from the original several times in an attempt to eliminate "yes" and "no" answers, which were not helpful. The evaluations are extremely valuable and several times have indicated changes that needed to be made in the LAMS program to make it more useful or easier to understand. They also are an aid to research as to outcomes of the program.

The Pretty Prize is awarded at the very end of the session. Names are written on small slips of paper and dropped in a bag at sign-in, and one name is drawn at the end of the session. Be sure to ask if everyone has entered their name for the drawing. It is really a door prize to encourage attendance and increase self-esteem. The "Pretty Prize" name is descriptive, as it includes one or two items such as perfume, bath supplies, fingernail polish, jewelry, or a watch—something to make the winner feel "special"—as well as sample items such as soaps, lotions, or shampoo. All the things are placed in a lunch bag or similar size container and stapled at the top. Items are sometimes donated or may have to be purchased. If the group contains both men and women, bags should be prepared for both. Men's bags may contain cologne, shaving lotion and other shaving supplies, watches, or other small toiletries, as well as appropriate samples. The winner opens the bag and shows the group what is inside, so all can share in the excitement. Occasionally, two or three names are drawn if special holiday items are being given.

When there is time, close each session with the Car Wash exercise. All group members and leaders assemble in two facing lines about two feet apart with approximately equal numbers on each side. One person at a time, from alternating sides, goes down the middle; others may pat them on the back or give encouraging comments, such as "You look nice today," "Glad you could be here," or "You helped out a lot during the session." This continues until all have gone down the center aisle. This is a self-esteem-building exercise, one used in many types of support groups.

A graduation certificate is awarded upon completion of the series; one can be designed on a computer or by hand. An example is included at the end of this chapter. This is an important self-esteem builder, as many participants have never graduated from anything before. Pictures can be taken at that time—one to be given to the group member and one mounted on a graduate "honor roll." The graduation ceremony can be as elaborate as desired.

Two other forms are used when group members graduate. They are a questionnaire for the participant to complete and another to be given to the caseworker or other person who sent them to the group, if that is why they are there. The caseworker returns the questionnaire to the facilitator after completion. They are similar in content and have several of the same questions. Comparing the answers helps to evaluate the participants' views of changes made through attending LAMS, as well as what changes the caseworkers observe during their clients' attendance. During the five years these have been used, the two forms have been mostly in agreement as to changes made or recognized. Changes could be made in the questions asked in order to make them relevant to your program. These forms are also included in this chapter, and research analysis of the answers is included in Dr. Berry's study in the appendix.

GENERAL INSTRUCTIONS FOR FACILITATORS

Each week, prior to the session meeting, the facilitator should:

- Set up the room, if necessary.
- Write on the board: "LAMS," followed by the week number of the session, the topic for the week, and the date. This information is needed for completion of the evaluation forms.

- Arrange sign-in materials: name tags, notebook or paper for sign-in, pens and markers, slips of paper to register for the Pretty Prize, bag to hold registrations. A stuffed lamb toy can also be placed there as a "mascot."
- Prepare Pretty Prize bag with health or beauty products for men or women, both masculine and feminine prize bags if you have a mixed group.
- Gather materials needed as listed in each weekly introduction.
- If food is served, be sure cups, plates or bowls, and utensils are available.

Facilitators can add or delete games or activities for the ones specified, depending on the size and makeup of the group. The activities should be tied to the theme for the week even though participants may not recognize their purpose at first. The ones included in this book are "survivors" of much trial and error; unsuccessful choices were eliminated. Any local library should be able to provide additional material.

When crafts are included, the facilitator should practice the craft first and make a sample item for the group members to refer to if they need help or ideas. Remember not to attempt something that is too difficult; you are trying to build successes, not failures. Everyone should have something to be proud of at the end of the session. All written materials should be read aloud to accommodate any group members with reading difficulties. Quizzes and questionnaires should be read orally, one question at a time, before discussion. The facilitator, an assistant, or another group member should provide extra help to anyone who cannot read or write. With these adaptations, the LAMS program can be successfully completed by everyone, even those who are mentally, physically, or educationally challenged.

Do not hesitate to skip parts of a session or change the time allowed if the group is discussing something that is important to them. They can often learn more from each other than could be taught by facilitators interrupting them to continue the stated agenda.

Above all, LAMS should be an enjoyable experience. Many participants were told they must attend the group; they did not come because they wanted to. They do not want to hear a lecture or a sermon. Listen to what group members have to say, too. Make the participants want to come back because it was interesting and they felt good about being there. Talk about local news, what group members have been doing, the weather, anything—just do not be *boring*.

LAMS facilitators do not have to be teachers or therapists, and they do not have to be perfect examples. It is impossible to *make* group members change; they have to *want* to change, and they have to have the information to show them *how* to change. The LAMS curriculum provides the information needed, but the facilitator must convey it in the most interesting way possible for the program to be effective.

PRE-LAMS QUESTIONNAIRE

Name _____

Date _____

1. What did you never have as a child that you wanted?

2. What have you always wanted to do that you have never done?

3. What would you most like to have that you do not have now?

4. What do you dislike the most about yourself?

5. What do you like the most about yourself?

6. How do you feel about your life? Happy? Sad? Angry? Do you feel as if life just "happens" to you, and you are not in control?

7. What things do you do to feel better about yourself and your life?

8. How would you most like to change your life right now?

9. How would you like to change your looks?

10. What person has changed your life the most? How did he or she change it?

11. Would you like to be "just like" someone else? Who? Why?

12. What do you do for fun by yourself or with your family?

13. What is one thing you have always wanted to know about or learn to do?

14. When you were a child, what did you want to be when you grew up?

15. What do you want most for your child/children when he or she/ they grow up?

16. What do you want your life to be like five years from now?

LAMS WEEKLY EVALUATION

Week # _____
Date _____

1. What was the most helpful thing you learned today? _____

_____

_____

2. Do you feel you learned something about the topic for the week, and could you understand everything that was presented?
yes _____ no _____   yes _____ no _____

3. Was there anything you did NOT like about the lesson?
yes _____ no _____

How could we change the lesson so you would have liked it better? _____

_____

4. What could have been added to the session today to make it more helpful? _____

_____

_____

5. What changes are you making in your life as a result of what you have learned in LAMS? _____

_____

_____

_____

LAMS GRADUATION QUESTIONNAIRE
FOR GROUP MEMBER

Name _____

Date _____

1. Have you received any kind of professional counseling or therapy other than this group experience? yes _____ no _____
   If yes, when and where? _____

2. As a child, were you a victim of:
   physical abuse _____
   emotional abuse _____
   neglect _____
   incest (sexual abuse by a relative) _____
   rape (nonrelative) _____

3. As an adult, have you been a victim of:
   spousal abuse _____
   rape or sexual abuse (nonrelative) _____

4. Have you made new friends in the LAMS group?
   yes _____ no _____ How many? _____

5. Have you talked on the phone or visited other LAMS group members between sessions? yes _____ no _____
   How many members? _____

6. Has your appearance changed any since you joined LAMS?
   yes _____ no _____ If yes, how? _____

   _____

7. Did you learn new ways to solve problems or make decisions while attending LAMS? _____

   _____

8. Do you think before you act more often now than before you attended LAMS? _____

_____

9. Do you now feel that you have choices and you are more in control of your life? _____

_____

10. Do you think you are more assertive (can ask reasonably for what you want and need) now than before?

   yes _____ no _____ If yes, how? _____

_____

11. Have you done anything on your own recently that you would have been afraid to do before attending LAMS?

   yes _____ no _____ If yes, what? _____

_____

12. Do you feel you are a better parent now than before you began attending LAMS? yes _____ no _____ If yes, how? _____

_____

13. The parts of the LAMS group experience that helped me the most were:

   Learning how what happened in the past affects
   the present _____

   Learning to identify and accept my feelings _____

   Learning how to make choices that will change my life _____

   Learning to be assertive, not passive or aggressive _____

   Learning practical skills, such as making healthier meals
   or budgeting my money _____

Learning how to get more education _____

Experiencing warm relationships in the group _____

Other: _____

14. I wish we had learned more about _____

_____

15. The one thing I learned that was the most important to me was

_____

Any other comments? _____

_____

If the group member was referred by someone—caseworker, social worker, etc.—the referring person should fill out the following form after the client's completion of the LAMS program. The facilitator completes the information on the top three lines before giving it to the referring person. After completion, the form should be returned to the facilitator for comparison with the client's responses to be sure changes are noted both by the graduate and the referring person.

Group member's name _____

Referred by _____

Graduation date _____

POST-LAMS QUESTIONNAIRE

You referred the above person to the LAMS program. Please answer the following questions about changes you may have observed since his or her participation, and return this questionnaire to the Facilitator, _____, as soon as possible.

Thank you!

1. Do you feel that your client is still as socially isolated since attending LAMS? yes _____ no _____

2. Does your client seek help from others more now than before attending LAMS? yes _____ no _____

3. Has your client learned to solve problems or make better decisions since attending LAMS? yes _____ no _____

   Any examples? _____

   _____

4. Has your client improved in appearance since attending LAMS? yes _____ no _____ How? _____

   _____

5. Have you seen any indication of improved self-esteem? yes _____ no _____ What? _____

   _____

6. Is your client more assertive than before attending LAMS?
   yes _____ no _____

7. Is your client more independent than before attending LAMS?
   yes _____ no _____ How has this been shown? _____

   _____

8. Do you feel that the LAMS group has helped your client make life
   changes? yes _____ no _____ Examples: _____

   _____

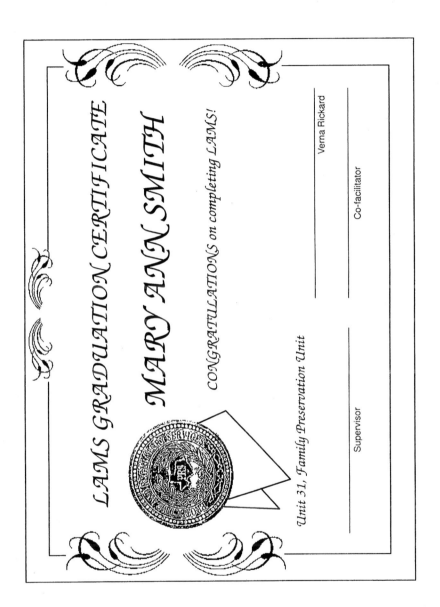

LAMS GRADUATION CERTIFICATE

MARY ANN SMITH

CONGRATULATIONS on completing LAMS!

Unit 31, Family Preservation Unit

_____
Supervisor

_____
Verna Rickard
Co-facilitator

Chapter 3

Week One: My Self

Goals for the Week Are:

1. To promote group interaction through "When I" game
2. To complete "Choices" questionnaire and discuss
3. To compare brain and computer
4. To learn how choices are made
5. To learn that life does not just "happen" to you

Materials Needed:

A Participant Handbook for each group member
Pens, felt-tip markers, and notebook or paper for sign-in
Name tags
Pencils for participants
Questions for "When I" game
Chalkboard, flip chart, or large pad of drawing paper (could have
   a predrawn, four-drawer file cabinet)
Pretty Prize(s)

My Self week is the basis for the entire LAMS program. Its main premise is that life is made up of choices, good and bad. Many participants have made bad choices or no choices at all, and life has just "happened" to them; they feel they have no control. This session will point out that many life experiences thought of as "happenings" were really choices. Those events could have been changed by making the right decisions in the beginning and following through. Bad choices can be recognized, acknowledged, and many times changed. Mistakes are not something to be ashamed of, rather something to learn from. Group members can learn to live their lives by *choice*, not by *chance*.

Begin the session with introductions and a short explanation of the LAMS program if there are new members. Explain that LAMS is a fifteen-week program designed to help them feel better about themselves and their lives, help them learn to make better choices, get along with others, and find out how what happened to them in the past affects what they are doing now. They will learn many practical skills, find out how to get more education, how to be healthier, and how to take time for themselves.

Ask everyone to turn to Week One in their handbooks and read the Affirmation in unison. Every weekly session begins with an Affirmation. This helps participants form new thought patterns that are positive instead of negative. Many have never succeeded at anything they have attempted and are afraid to try again. Their self-talk tells them they will never be any different; they are doomed to failure. LAMS constantly tells them that they *can* achieve, that they are important, and that they are worthwhile individuals. The facilitator should then read "Choices" and "I'm OK" aloud; participants can follow along in their books.

The next activity, the "When I" game, is a self-revealing series of questions that helps the participants get acquainted and shows the facilitator any special needs which should be addressed. The questions should be printed on 3-by-5 cards in advance, if they are to be passed around the group, or questions can be asked from the list by the facilitator, one at a time to each participant. The game moves faster if the questions are asked by the leaders, especially if the group is fairly large.

The second activity, the "Choices" questionnaire, is for discussion only. It reveals past and present decisions and the group members' attitudes about themselves and their families. All the questions should be read aloud and completed as a group so anyone with reading difficulties is able to participate. Discuss the answers after all are completed, but only in general. Do not ask each member for his or her response; some may not wish to reveal their answers.

The third and most important part of this week's session explains how choices are made. It compares the brain to a computer in terms of how much information can be stored and how bits from different areas can be "pulled up" as needed. Choices are made constantly. Things do not just "happen"; they are the result of those choices. The facilitator may want to prepare a poster board with a picture of a four-drawer file cabinet and attach self-stick notes for what is learned and kept in each drawer. The first drawer contains what was learned as a baby, the second, as a preschooler, the third what was learned in school, and the fourth all the other things learned—reactions, opinions, ideas, hopes, fears, self-image, prejudices, and what is seen as right and wrong. This file cabinet can also be drawn on a chalkboard or flip chart if desired. Read through the information on making choices before attempting to teach it. Examples can be changed according to the makeup of the group, if desired. Be sure to ask for examples of choices group members made since they woke up this morning (e.g., turn off the alarm, get out of bed), so you can be sure everyone understands the material.

Since the LAMS program is designed so that each week is independent and open ended, members may begin any week and attend until that week comes around again (or at least ten weeks, if ill, etc.). If there are any participants graduating during this session, a certificate of completion should be given and pictures taken. The certificate can be designed using computer templates or by hand. It is important to give some type of recognition, as it is an important occasion. Many group members have never graduated from anything before and are proud of their accomplishment. Some past participants have "dressed up" in special clothing for their graduation. The ceremony can be held at any point in the session or during break and can be as elaborate as you wish. Two instant camera pictures are taken, one for the participant and one to be mounted on a poster board "Graduate Honor Roll."

Close with evaluations and the Pretty Prize drawing; do the Car Wash exercise if there is time. These are all explained in the following material.

WEEK ONE: MY SELF

• Registration should be completed before time for class to begin. Pass out Participant Handbooks to any new group members. Include the Pre-LAMS Questionnaire if one is used and explain that it is to be handed in at the end of the session.

• Introduce facilitator(s) and briefly explain the LAMS program. Housekeeping issues should be addressed (location of bathrooms, smoking, break, etc.). Make any special announcements, especially if there is no session the following week due to a holiday or other reason. (Time: 5 minutes.)

• Read the Affirmation aloud, in unison; group members should use the Participant Handbook. (Time: 5 minutes.)

> I am important.
> What I say is important.
> What I think is important.
> What I do is important,
> To myself and those around me.
> I choose to be the best, most caring, accepting, and
> understanding person I can be.

• Facilitator should read aloud the "Making Choices" reading. Participants should follow along in their books. All material is read aloud, as some group members may have reading difficulties. (Time: 5 minutes.)

MAKING CHOICES

You may feel that a lot of things have just "happened" to you in your life. Really, *you* have made them happen. Your past choices have put you where you are today.

When you learn how to make the right choices, you can choose what you want your life to be like and change what it is like now.

You can choose to live your life by *choice*, not by *chance*.

• Facilitator should read aloud the "I'm OK" readings. Participants should follow along in their handbooks. (Time: 3 minutes.)

I'M OK

I'm really OK. I will learn to like myself. I will do nice things for myself, or by myself. I will treat myself to things I really want to do, such as read a book or go for a walk. I don't have to do what other people want me to do all of the time. I am still "me" inside, even if I am a mother or father, a child to my own parents, a wife or girlfriend, or a husband or boyfriend. I have needs of my own, and time I spend alone helps me to understand who I am. I do not have to like everybody, and everybody does not have to like me. I will change myself, even though I cannot change others. I will say good things to myself and tell myself I am a good person. This may be hard because I do not always feel like those things are true. I will think about what I *can* do, not what I *cannot* do. I will be good to my body by eating right and taking care of myself, so I will feel better and look better. I will be nice to others and say nice things to them so they will like themselves better, too. I will enjoy being the great person that I am!

• Introduce the self-revealing game, "When I." Questions can be copied to 3-by-5 cards and passed around the circle, or the facilitator can ask them one at a time, to each group member. More or different questions can be added if you choose. They are good discussion starters, so allow time between questions for comments from other participants. If you cannot finish all the questions in the allotted time, stop and go on to the next activity. (Time: 15 minutes.)

"WHEN I" GAME QUESTIONS

When I make a mistake, I _____
When I get angry, I _____
I think men are _____
When I think of my father, I _____
The thing I would most like to buy for my house is

_____

When I think of my mother, I _____

I like to _____
When I am around men, I _____
The thing that makes me happiest is _____
The worst thing that could happen to me would be
_____
When I am around women, I _____
I know I should _____
When I was a child, I always wanted _____
Women annoy me when they _____
When people criticize me, I _____
I can't understand why _____
Men annoy me when they _____
I have always wanted to _____
When I want to have fun, I _____
The most important thing about childhood is
_____
I feel as if life _____
When I think about my ideal job, I _____
It makes me angry when _____
When I can't quiet a crying baby, I _____
In five years, I want to _____
My favorite food is _____
I don't know why _____
When I think of my childhood family, I _____
Men's chores should include _____
It makes me cry when I _____
When someone I don't know calls me a "broad," or a
    "chick," or "sweetie," I _____
When I meet someone new, I _____
I have always wanted to learn how to _____
If I had more money, I would _____
If I could have anything I wished for, it would be
_____
I get depressed when I _____
An attractive man (or woman) to me is _____
Women are _____
If I could undo something that has happened to me, it
    would be _____

When I was little, I wanted to grow up to be a

_____

My friends think that I _____
When I think of my favorite place, it is _____
The thing about me I would most like to change is

_____

I'm sorry I _____
When I'm happy, I _____
I feel helpless when I _____
I feel afraid when I _____
When I am alone, I _____
When I am in a large group, I _____
I feel sad when I _____
I get jealous when _____
My favorite season of the year is _____
I feel unwanted when I _____
I feel special when I _____
My favorite color is _____
When people in my family argue, I _____
The person who has most influenced my life is

_____

When I was a child, I felt closest to _____
My favorite class when I was in school was

_____

When I was bad as a child, my parents _____

• Complete the "Choices" Questionnaire in the Participant Handbook. All questions should be read aloud and completed as a group. There is no scoring; this is for self-information only. After the questions are completed, discuss them one by one. Do not ask for individual answers; allow group members to respond if they wish. (Time: 30 minutes.)

CHOICES QUESTIONNAIRE

1. Is your life better than your mother's or father's was?

   Yes _____ No _____ Undecided _____

2. Do you think your life will be better five years from now?

   Yes _____ No _____ Undecided _____

3. Do you think your children will have a better life than you have had?

   Yes _____ No _____ Undecided _____

4. Would your life be different today if you had:

Different parents?	Y____ N____ U____
More education?	Y____ N____ U____
Gotten involved with someone else?	Y____ N____ U____
Not had children at a young age?	Y____ N____ U____
More money?	Y____ N____ U____

5. Has your life changed through:

Decisions *you* made?	Y____ N____ U____
Decisions *others* made for you?	Y____ N____ U____
Things that just happened?	Y____ N____ U____

6. Most of the time, are you doing what:

You want to do?	Y____ N____ U____
Others want you to do?	Y____ N____ U____

7. Have you ever had a substance abuse problem?   Y____ N____ U____

8. Do you think women have more self-control than men?   Y____ N____ U____

9. Do you believe you can change the
   person you have a relationship with? Y____ N____ U____

10. Do you have to have a man/woman
    in your life to be happy? Y____ N____ U____

11. What things do you do to get your own way in a disagreement
    with your mate?

    Check all that apply:

    Argue ____

    Reason ____

    Pout ____

    Withhold sex ____

    Trick him or her ____

    Threaten to leave ____

12. Not counting regular bills or expenses, how much money would
    you spend without talking it over with your mate?

    $10-$20 ____

    $20-$50 ____

    $50-$100 ____

    More? ____

13. Which of these things do you usually do for your mate?

    Buy clothing? ____

    Wash clothing? ____

    Iron or put away clothing? ____

    Cook meals? ____

    Entertain his or her family or friends? ____

    Wait on him or her? ____

    Make medical or other appointments? ____

14. How well could your mate get along without you:

    For everyday needs?   Very well ____ OK ____   Not at all ____

    Emotionally?   ____   ____   ____

    Financially?   ____   ____   ____

    Sexually?   ____   ____   ____

15. How well could your family manage without you for a few days?

    Very well _____ OK _____ Not at all _____

16. How would you feel if they did well without you for that time?

    Awful, not needed _____ OK _____ Makes no difference _____

17. Who decides:

    What you watch on TV?   You ____ Mate ____ Kids ____

    What is for dinner?   ____   ____   ____

    Who your friends are?   ____   ____   ____

18. How often do your needs come before those of your family?

    Sometimes _____ Always _____ Never _____

19. Do you think men and women have equal opportunities:

    At work?   Yes _____   No _____

    At home?   _____   _____

20. If you don't work now, would you go to work if you could get affordable daycare?

    Yes _____ No _____

21. Do you sometimes do things yourself because you feel only you can do things the right way?

    Yes _____ No _____

22. Do you sometimes feel that life just "happens" to you and you have no control?

    Yes _____ No _____

23. Do you feel that you have more problems than most people?

    Yes _____ No _____

24. Check one—Would you say that your life is generally:

    The best? _____

    Better than most? _____

    About average? _____

    Worse than most? _____

    The pits? _____

• Facilitator announces time for a break. Food should be served buffet style. Older children may eat in the nursery, or parents may bring them to the classroom. Parents may want to check on their children during break. (Time: 30 minutes.)

• Facilitator presents information on similarities between brain and computer. A good reference book for this section is *Choices*, by Saul Helmstetter (Pocket Books, 1989). Reading this book will provide a good overview of how and why certain choices are made. (Time: 45 minutes.)

BRAIN AND COMPUTER

Your brain is similar to a computer. Computers store large quantities of information and keep all of that information in order. Your brain does the same thing. Everything that is fed into a computer is registered there, regardless of whether it is put in yesterday, today, or tomorrow. Computers don't "forget" things, even though what they know may not be on the screen and available to be read all the time. The same thing happens with your memory. Everything is there. Sometimes you may have covered something up so you don't *have* to remember it, but it is still there somewhere. The main difference is that something can be erased from a computer but not from your brain, except possibly from some accidentally caused brain damage. All that information can be called up at any time.

Here is a picture of a big, four-drawer file cabinet (draw one on the board, or use a predrawn one). In the top drawer (point to it) are all the new skills you learned as a baby, such as how to eat and drink, how to crawl, and even how to walk. (Ask group members to call out other skills.) Some other examples are how to recognize Mom, Dad, and other caretakers, know and respond to your own name, and identify animals and the sounds they make. Since you have grown up, you do not have to tell your body how to walk across the room. At one time, when you were first learning to walk, you had to think about how to hold your body, how to move your legs and feet, and how to keep your balance. Now you eat without thinking, talk easily, and get through your day with little thought to those basic skills. They are all easier, but only after a lot of practice.

Later on (point to the second drawer), you made another file in your brain to hold what you learned in your preschool years. (Ask group members for examples.) In that drawer, you filed away how to go to the bathroom instead of wearing diapers, how to play with other children, how to tie your shoes, how to identify what you saw in your world, how to say "no" and be your own person, and millions of other pieces of information you needed to live your life.

The third drawer (point to it) contains what you learned in school, such as how to read and write. What else did you learn in school? (Have them call out what they learned, then the facilitator should add other skills not already identified.) You used those basic skills as building blocks to learn more about your world.

In the fourth drawer (point to it), you stored away all of your other experiences—what happened to you before, while, or since you were in school. These might include your reactions to what people said to you, whether good or bad. This drawer would contain your opinions and ideas, your hopes and fears, and how you feel about yourself now. It would include your prejudices and what you think is right or wrong.

Of course your brain is much more complicated than a computer; this is only an example. You do not really have file cabinets to store the information, but it *is* all there someplace, filed away even when you aren't using it. Every time you make a decision or a choice, you get information out of one or more, and maybe even *all* of those drawers. Your life is not just "happening" to you; you are *choosing* your own path.

Think about how you make decisions. You make them all day, every day. Your first choice of the day may be how quickly you get up when the alarm goes off or when you wake up and know you must get out of bed. Do you push the "snooze" button or close your eyes for "just another minute" of sleep? Look back at those file drawers. How do you know how to reach for the clock? How do you know what the "snooze" button is or what it is for? Why do you feel that you must have another minute of sleep? Did your mother let you stay in bed for a while after she first called you, and were you sure she would come back and call you again? Is there somebody with you now that you are sure will wake you up if you go back to sleep? Look in the last drawer—the one with your beliefs and ideas in it. If you don't get your kids off to school, will you hear your mother in your head telling you that you are a poor parent and a bad person? Will you feel you are not being responsible if you do not get to your doctor appointment or to work? Or did your care-takers skip such obligations regularly when you were a child? How did you learn to tell time in the first place?

As you can see, those file drawers and that computer in your head can have a big influence on how you act today and on what choices you make for yourself. You, alone, are not making those choices; in fact—much of the time—you do not even recognize that they *are* choices.

Now we will go on to a more difficult choice. Suppose you need money for groceries to feed your children. You are not due to get any money for at least a week. What kind of decisions could you make, and why would you make them?

Your first choice might be not to buy groceries at all. Why would you do that? You and your family are hungry, but you can borrow or beg some food from family or friends. How you feel about those people, and how they feel about you, might affect that choice. Maybe you have run out of food before and asked your family for help, and you remember they said that they would not help you again. Maybe you have asked the neighbors for help many times, also. You may also have too much pride (remembered from your files) to ask anyone for help even if you think they might help you.

Now think of other possible ways to get money. You do not have a job, so that is not a choice. If you could get a job, you would not get money right away. Maybe you could *steal* some money? Now you get input from your files again. How do you feel about stealing? Do you feel it is wrong? (moral teaching, maybe from church as a child) Do you only fear getting caught by the police? (maybe from knowing someone who got arrested) How did your parents feel about stealing? (maybe they did it all the time, so it was okay, or maybe they would have *never* stolen for any reason) Would you be embarrassed if your friends found out you stole something? After considering everything in your file drawers, your choice is made in seconds. We never think about the memories behind the choices we make, any more than we think about what we have to do to walk across the room.

Your final choice made, in order to get food, may be to go to the nearest church that you know has a free food program, tell them what your problem is, and get help there. That is morally okay; you will not get arrested or be embarrassed in front of your friends; your parents will not be unhappy with you, and your children will get food.

That choice takes information out of many of your file drawers. You have to know how to get to the church, what days they give out food, what time of day to go, how to read the name of the church, and how to fill out the application form. Maybe you had to call the church first, before you went, to find out what you needed to know. After you get the food, you have to know how to get back home, how to prepare it, and even how to pick up the fork or spoon to get it into your mouth. And you thought making choices was *simple*!

Can any of you think of some examples of choices you have made already today? (Carry through suggestions from start to finish—how they made the choice they made; take several if you have time.)

From now on, do not make all of your choices without thinking about them. What you buy at the grocery store is a choice. You can spend all of your money on junk food and be out of money by next week, or you can choose to shop sensibly, buy things that stretch your money, and have some left at the end of the month. That is a *choice*; it does not just *happen*. If you do not pay the rent, you are *choosing* to possibly be evicted. If you do not want to be evicted, you would have to make a different choice, such as going to get help, trying to work something out with your landlord, getting help from a friend, or moving somewhere else you could afford. Life does not just *happen* to you; the choices you make are your own, and life just follows along. If you take drugs, you may become an addict. If you drink heavily, you will probably get drunk. Everything you do has a result, or a consequence, and if you think about those consequences *before* you make your choices, your life will be in *your* control.

This is what you will be learning in LAMS every week—how you can be in charge of your life. Many of you did not learn how to do this at home; some of you may not have thought it was *possible* to be in control. Some people say they cannot do it because of what happened to them as children, or because everyone dislikes them, or they do not have much education, or they are only twenty-one years old and have three children. These are just excuses—you *can* learn to be in charge; in fact, you have already learned today how and why you make the choices you make and how to put more thought into them. You have learned that nothing "out there" controls you—you do it yourself.

• Distribute evaluation forms; have pencils available. Names are optional. They can leave them facedown on one of the tables. (Time: 5 minutes.)

• Complete Pretty Prize drawing. Be sure everyone put their name in the bag. The facilitator, a guest, or group member can draw the name for the prize. Winner must show contents to the others. The same person cannot win two weeks in succession. This is a *very* popular part of the session! (Time: 5 minutes.)

• Car Wash is a self-esteem building activity. Have group members divide equally into two facing lines, about three feet apart. One person at a time, from alternate lines, proceeds down the middle to the other end. Every person on each side pats him/her on the back and gives positive affirmations, such as, "Glad you were here," "You look nice today," etc. Be sure participants do not mind being touched; otherwise, use only verbal affirmations. (Due to time and space, this is difficult to do weekly, but do it when possible as a closing exercise.) (Time: 5 minutes.)

Chapter 4

Week Two: My Attitude

Goals for the Week Are:

1. To learn differences between positive and negative attitudes
2. To learn the risks of rejection
3. To role-play positive and negative attitudes

Materials Needed:

A Participant Handbook for each group member
Pens, felt-tip markers, and paper or notebook for sign-in
Name tags
Pencils for participants
Paper for group to list positives and negatives about themselves
Chalkboard, flip chart, or large pad of drawing paper
Pretty Prize(s)

Attitude week illustrates the importance of thinking positively, rather than negatively. It teaches participants how to think positively about themselves and shows how a positive attitude affects others. Group members role-play differences in attitude and learn that they should talk to themselves as a friend, not an enemy, because what they *think* controls how they *feel*.

The facilitator should begin by asking group members to turn to Week Two in their handbooks; then the Affirmation is read aloud, in unison. "Attitude Is Contagious" should then be read aloud by the leader, with participants following along in their handbooks. "Love and the Cabbie" is another good article on attitude to read to the group (Canfield and Wells, 1976).

Ask group members to list positives and negatives about themselves; then have them call out some of them to be written on the board or flip chart.

The game, "You've Got It—I Want It," illustrates very well the object of this week's lesson on attitude. Leaders should demonstrate how to play the game before asking the others to begin. Use various techniques to get your way, overacting if necessary—begging, pleading, getting mad, making your partner feel guilty—but do not tell the group the object of the game, which is to demonstrate how people act in a disagreement. The role-plays can be done by twos, with everyone watching, or all at once if it is a large group. They are excellent for teaching concepts and usually cause lots of laughter. Most participants enjoy role-plays, and some really get into the spirit of the game. After everyone has had a turn, explain that they have just illustrated how people try to get their own way and how attitudes change during these attempts. This activity is a good lead-in for the discussion of self-talk and having a good self-concept.

Continue with role-plays of positive and negative attitudes, of being an optimist instead of a pessimist. Finally, talk about how those persons closest to an individual—his or her mate, children, or family—can upset him or her the most because he or she values their opinion and wants it to be positive.

Close as usual with evaluations, the Pretty Prize drawing, and the Car Wash exercise if time allows.

WEEK TWO: MY ATTITUDE

• Register all new members and give each a Participant Handbook and Pre-LAMS Questionnaire to be completed and handed in at the end of the session.

• Introduce facilitator(s), briefly explain the LAMS program, and address housekeeping issues. (Time: 5 minutes.)

• Read Affirmation aloud, in unison. Participants should read from their handbooks. (Time: 5 minutes.)

I choose to have a good attitude.
I will see life as good.
I will be myself and not hide behind a mask.
I will do everything I can to see the best in myself
    and others around me.

• Read aloud, "Attitude Is Contagious." (Time: 5 minutes.)

ATTITUDE IS CONTAGIOUS

Have you ever had a *really* bad day—one when everything you did was wrong? It all started when you kicked the edge of the door on the way to the bathroom; what you wanted to wear was dirty; and the hot water was cold. By the time you got to the kitchen you were cross and out of sorts. Your children made you angry because they were slow getting to the table for breakfast. Your husband could not find what he needed for work, and you were *not* in the mood to help him look for it. The school bus was early, and the kids were late. Your good-bye as they went out the door was angry and frustrated.

What about *their* day? How did your attitude affect them? Probably they were short-tempered with their friends, sarcastic when answering their teachers, and spoiling for an argument until later in the day, when the effects of your mood wore off.

Now think of the opposite. What about a *great* day? You bounced out of bed, the sun was shining, and you looked forward to your trip to the store. You complimented your teenaged daughter on her choice of clothing, telling her how nice she looked. You told your son he had done a really good job cleaning up the yard, and let your husband know you especially liked his new tie. All the family responded to your good mood, being positive themselves. You smiled at the kids when they left for school and told them you loved them.

What about the rest of their day? Exactly. *Your* attitude changed *their* attitude. They gave compliments to their friends, were pleasant to their teachers, and were nicer to everyone they met.

Remember that "glow" you feel for hours after someone tells you how nice you look or how pretty your shirt is? What about the opposite—when the checker at the grocery store is rude and disagreeable? You often respond in the same manner. We all need to remember that it costs nothing extra to be kind and polite to others, and hopefully, they will pass it on to everyone they meet later in the day. Not only colds are contagious—attitude is too!

Discuss how positive attitudes change the behavior of others, as well as yourself. (Time: 5 minutes.)

• Pass out paper and pencils and have group members list five positive and five negative things about themselves. After four minutes ask which was harder. (positive) Ask if anyone wants to share his or her list. (Time: 5 minutes.)

• Ask participants to call out positive attitudes. List these on a chalkboard or large pad of paper. (I am happy, pretty, smart, loved.) Then list negatives. (I am afraid, dumb, unemployable, ugly.) Discuss how your attitude affects how you feel about yourself and others. (Time: 15 minutes.)

• Begin the exercise, "You've Got It—I Want It." This exercise is based on one developed by John O. Stevens, which appeared in *Awareness*, pp. 112-113.

Directions:

• Instruct group members to count off in twos. Explain the following rules (Time: 10 minutes):

I want you to play a game called, "You've Got It—I Want It." Imagine that those with the number "1" have, and want very much to keep, something that the "2s" want very badly. Think what it might be: clothing, jewelry, a car, anything. "2s" might start off by saying, "I want it," and "1s" answer, "I won't give it to you." Continue by saying anything you think might work to get it for yourself (if you're a "2") or hang onto it (if you're a "1"). (Demonstrate with your co-facilitator or a volunteer.) Have everyone do this at the same time. (After two to three minutes, switch roles and repeat the process.)

What happened? . . . (*Ellipses indicate responses from group members.*) How did you try to get it? . . . (beg, reason, bribe, demand, threaten, get angry, make partner feel guilty) What did your partner say to keep the item? . . . How did you feel when you told your partner you weren't giving it up? . . . (powerful, in charge, angry, guilty) Did you want to give it up just to make peace or to please the other person? . . .

This is not just a game; it brings out some of the ways you behave when you are in an argument or when you want to get your own way. Think about how you acted—if you got mad or if you just wanted to give in and get it over with. What kind of an attitude do you have when this is real? . . .

• Lead a discussion about self-talk. Begin with the introduction below. (Time: 20 minutes.)

Have you ever heard a little voice in your head talking to you? . . . No, I do not mean that I think you are crazy. I am talking about the voice that says, "Stupid, why did you say that? You never can keep your mouth shut!" or "There you go again, always making mistakes." That little voice is called "self-talk." Your mind does it even while your body is doing something else. If what you hear in your head is positive—telling you that you are a good person—you probably feel good about yourself. If all you hear is that you are bad, you probably feel depressed and down. How you *think* controls how you *feel*.

Think about how you talk to yourself. Would you say those hurtful words to a friend? If not, how can you learn to love yourself and forgive yourself for making mistakes? . . . (Tell yourself you are a great person.)

We begin each LAMS session with an *Affirmation*, something to help you focus on positives not negatives. Listen to what you hear in your head. If your little voice never says anything good, teach it something new. If you always hear that you are "stupid," stop and think where that came from. Did your parents say that, and did you think it was true then? Is it true *now*? If not, tell yourself you are smart, and you can learn to do anything. Until you *think* you can, you *cannot*. Changing what that little voice says is hard, but with practice you can do it.

• Announce time for a break and food. Children may eat with adults if desired. (Time: 30 minutes.)

• What do you think of you? Listen to this quote by John Powell, from his book, *Why Am I Afraid to Love?*: "But, if I tell you who I am, you may not like who I am, and it is all I have." What do you think he means? . . . (If everyone knew all the bad things about him, they would reject him.)

How many of you sometimes put on a mask or a false front when dealing with other people? . . . Do you ever pretend to be what someone else wants you to be? . . . If you are with a group of people who say things that make you feel uncomfortable, do you act as if you agree, just to be liked? . . . Do you feel that if someone knew all of your weaknesses and secret fears they would not like you? . . . That is exactly what John Powell is saying in that quote. It is a risk to go out on a limb and really be yourself—what if the other person does not like you for who you really are? If you find yourself living only for somebody else, you are not being true to yourself and what you can be. And that person cannot really be somebody to love if he or she cannot accept you for who you are. That person is not somebody you need in your life if you have to wear a mask in order to be loved, or even liked, by him or her. It is tiring to have to pretend all the time—you have to laugh at things that are not funny to you and try to remember all of the stories about yourself that were not really true.

Have you ever told someone about yourself and then been hurt because they would not listen and accept you for who you are?. . . Do you think it is too scary to be yourself and not be what somebody else wants you to be? . . .

I do not mean that you should bare your soul to everyone you meet in the grocery store. I mean that you should be able to be yourself and still be accepted. You do not have to confess your deepest fears to casual acquaintances, but your attitudes and feelings should be respected, and you should not have to hide who you are. You are a very special person, different from everyone else in the world. You have your own thoughts, and feelings, and beliefs, and they are what make you *you*. Learn to love yourself and appreciate how you are different. You cannot love someone else until you feel that you are a valuable human being. If you feel as if you are a bad person you may put up with being abused or not protect your children if they are abused—you feel you deserve to be punished for being bad. You have to accept that certain things may have happened to you; you cannot change them now. You have to accept that you are not perfect and forgive yourself. Only then can you have the positive attitude you need to live a happier life, and only then can you be in charge of your own life. (Time: 10 minutes.)

• Pass a half-full glass of liquid around the group. When all have seen it, ask someone to tell you what they saw (half-full or half-empty—optimist or pessimist). Address the group with the following (Time: 5 minutes):

> Is your "glass of life" half-full or half-empty? . . . Are you a pessimist who sees most things as bad or an optimist who sees most things as good? . . . How would you feel about this glass of water (or whatever) if you were in the middle of the desert? Would you be glad for the small drink, or would you complain that it wasn't enough? . . . You can change your attitude by thinking more positively about yourself and your life.

• Ask for two volunteers for a Role-Play on positive and negative attitudes. Decide who will be the husband and who the wife. Spend about five minutes on each scenario. Change roles halfway through the time. (Time: 15 minutes.)

Scenario 1

"It is raining—for the fourth day of your vacation. You saved money all year to be able to go to the beach for a week with your three children. Now you are all in one room watching it rain."

> One possible positive is that they are getting to know one another better; they seldom get to spend time together as a family or to sleep late. Another is that they can visit nearby indoor places which might be interesting, like museums. Some negatives are that the kids will not stop fighting and yelling, they are wasting all the money they saved because they cannot enjoy the beach, and they could have stayed at home if they wanted to watch TV all day.

Scenario 2

"You were fired from your job today and have to come home and tell your mate what happened."

> One positive is that you always hated that job because it was too far away. Maybe you will be able to get a better one. Some negatives are that you cannot help pay bills, buy food, or contribute to the rent, which could lead to eviction.

Scenario 3

"You find $10,000 in a suitcase, but the name and address of the owner are inside. Should you keep it?"

> Some positives are that you may get a reward for giving it back, you will make the owner happy, and you will not feel guilty. The negatives are that you need the money for bills, there will probably be no reward offered, and you really want to keep it but would feel guilty since you know who the owner is.

Remember, optimists find *something good* in everything; pessimists find *little good* in anything. You can find something good in almost every situation if you look hard enough.

• Do you have a positive attitude? Who is it that can push your buttons and control your attitudes? . . . (mate, kids, family, friends) Usually those who are closest to us are the best at knowing what upsets us. Your children are always experts at knowing what upsets you the most—and at using that knowledge! Why is that true? . . . (because if you did not love them you would not care what they said or if they approved of what you thought) Teens are great at telling their parents, "Everybody else gets to stay out late, why can't I?" If you did not love them, you would not *care* what they did; they *could* stay out late.

Would you rather be around a positive person or a negative one? . . . Have you ever known someone that made you feel awful? . . . Have you ever known a person who never had a good thing to say about anyone or anything? . . . What is different about someone who makes you feel good? . . . (he or she has positive thoughts, a good attitude, gives compliments) Which kind of person do *you* try to be? . . . Your attitude is contagious; how you feel and act can affect all the people around you. If you have a bad day, pretty soon all the people in your family will be yelling at each other. You will see only the storms and not the rainbows. (Time: 15 minutes.)

• Distribute evaluation forms; have pencils available. Names are optional. Collect them facedown on one of the tables. (Time: 5 minutes.)

• Hold the Pretty Prize drawing. Be sure all group members are entered. The same person cannot win two weeks in succession. (Time: 5 minutes.)

• Do the Car Wash exercise (see closing of Week One for instructions) if time allows. (Time: 5 minutes.)

Chapter 5

Week Three: My Relationships

Goals for the Week Are:

1. To learn how difficult it is to tell someone exactly what you mean
2. To recognize and deal with anger
3. To realize that "I have a bad temper" is an excuse
4. To learn the meaning of passive, aggressive, and assertive behaviors and to role-play each
5. To reinforce positive attitude and behavior

Materials Needed:

A Participant Handbook for each group member
Pens, felt-tip markers, and paper or notebook for sign-in
Name tags
Pencils for participants
2 blank 3-by-5 index cards for each group member
Diagram cards, 3-by-5 index cards with geometric figures drawn ahead of time, from instructions for "Describe a Shape" exercise
Chalkboard, flip chart, or large pad of drawing paper
Pretty Prize(s)

This week is about relationships. Many participants have trouble getting along with others, and some may have anger-control problems. Group members should turn to Week Three in their handbooks and read the Affirmation aloud, along with the facilitator.

The "Mirrors" exercise, which follows the Affirmation, is best explained by demonstrating it in front of the class, possibly by the two leaders or two volunteers from the group. It emphasizes the importance of eye contact in communication. "Imitation Circle" is another activity that may be chosen if the group is large enough. The group members will be surprised when eventually everyone is doing the same thing.

"Describe a Shape," the next activity, illustrates how hard it is to tell someone else *exactly* what you mean. This can be very important in an argument or when telling children what is expected of them, for example, when asking them to "clean up your room." They may have a very different understanding of what that means than their parent. Read the instructions carefully before beginning to describe the shape; remember to be *very* specific.

Read aloud "Do You Have to Please?" and talk about how group members often lose their own identities when they always try to please others. Everyone is special and different, and trying to be what someone else wants you to be makes you feel as if there is something wrong with how you really are.

Group participants may have little knowledge of passive, aggressive, or assertive behaviors and often do not recognize the advantages of acting assertively. All three are explained in this session in very basic terms, and role-plays are done to illustrate each concept. Many participants recognize themselves as exhibiting passive or aggressive behaviors, and now realize those behaviors may complicate their lives. The pages on behavioral types are included in the Participant Handbook, so group members can follow along when the information is read by the facilitator.

The session continues with learning to recognize and control anger. This is a teachable skill. "I have a bad temper" is an *excuse* for blowing up, not a *reason*. Keeping anger bottled up inside is just as big a mistake; it can cause real physical symptoms. It is much better to express it a little at a time before it explodes.

The last part of the session reinforces week two's focus on positive thinking and how constant complaining can cause problems in getting along with others.

The session ends with the usual evaluations, Pretty Prize drawing, and Car Wash exercise.

WEEK THREE: MY RELATIONSHIPS

• Register all new members and give each a Participant Handbook and Pre-LAMS Questionnaire to be completed and handed in at the end of the session.

• Introduce facilitator(s) and briefly describe the LAMS program and discuss housekeeping issues. (Time: 5 minutes.)

• Read the Affirmation aloud, in unison, with participants reading from their handbooks. (Time: 5 minutes.)

> I choose to talk in a way that tells others what I am thinking
> and allows them to see the best in me.
> I choose to believe in others and help them to believe
> in themselves.
> I will appreciate others for who they are and not try
> to change them.
> I will learn to control my temper and treat others fairly.
> I will listen to others and consider their opinions,
> But I will choose to do what is right for *me*.

• Begin with the self-esteem exercises. Choose "Mirrors" (pp. 37-39) or "Imitation Circle," based on activities in *Action Speaks Louder: A Handbook of Structured Group Techniques*, by Remocker and Storch. (Time: 15 minutes.)

MIRRORS

Number off in twos for this exercise or have two volunteers do the exercise in front of the group.

Partners stand facing each other about three feet apart. Decide who will be the leader and who will follow. Look each other in the eye as continuously as possible while the leader moves any part of his or her body very slowly, and the partner tries to mirror the moves without breaking eye contact. After a few minutes, switch roles.

When finished, discuss whether it was difficult to maintain eye contact and how important it is to look at other people in order to communicate well.

IMITATION CIRCLE

This is an alternative exercise, if the group is too large to effectively present "Mirrors."

There must be at least ten people for this exercise to work. It also illustrates communication through the use of your body.

Sit in a circle. Each person pick one person within one-fourth of the group on your right. Nobody else is to know who you have chosen. At "go," imitate this person's body posture, expression, movements, noises, etc. Continue for several minutes. Most people are surprised that soon everyone is doing the same thing.

• The following exercise illustrates that what you say is not always what others hear. (Time: 35 minutes.)

DESCRIBE A SHAPE EXERCISE

Draw several geometric figures (see possible examples) on blank 3-by-5 file cards, one on each card. Distribute two blank 3-by-5 file cards and a pencil to each group member.

The facilitator picks one figure-card and describes the shape aloud, very precisely. (For example, one and one-half inches from the right side of the card, straight up three inches, one inch to the left, etc.) Group members listen and try to reproduce the shape on one of their blank cards. The leader cannot use gestures, only words, and cannot answer questions. On completion of the diagram, participants are asked to hold up their cards so the leader can see the results. Comments can be made that some are close, but no identification should be made of a correct copy. Then participants are asked to turn the same card over and redraw the diagram as the leader describes the shape again—this time with gestures and responses to questions from the group. Ask them to hold up their cards

Possible examples for "Describe a Shape" exercise:

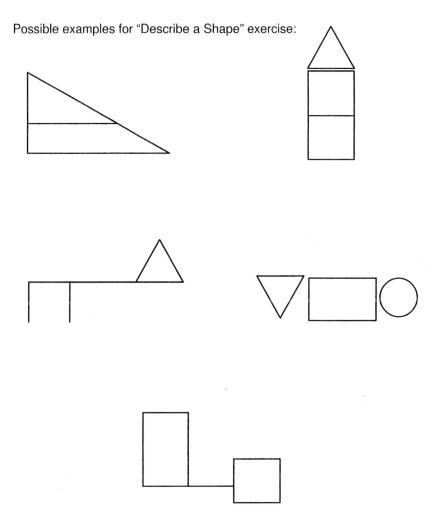

again with their new attempts. The facilitator then shows them the diagram they have been trying to copy. These copies should be much better, but few will be totally correct. Without much comment, repeat the exercise with a second diagram.

When everyone has completed the exercise, explain that they have just illustrated how hard it is to tell someone *exactly* what you mean. The speaker may think that what they are saying is perfectly clear; yet the listener is hearing something very different. Gestures and answers to questions make it more clear, but it is still hard to see what someone else is seeing or trying to explain.

This is what happens in an argument, when one person cannot understand why the other is unable to see his or her viewpoint. The same may happen when directions are given. Now they can see why their children have problems when they are told to "clean your room." What the parent says and what the child hears may be two different things. Directions are better given in small parts, so there is less chance for misunderstanding.

Allow time for discussion and questions.

• Announce time for a break and food. Children may eat with adults if desired. (Time: 30 minutes.)

• Read the following aloud; participants should follow along in their handbooks. (Time: 10 minutes.)

DO YOU HAVE TO PLEASE?

Are you a "pretzel" person? Are you somebody who has to bend and twist to please others? Many people, women especially, were raised to believe that they need to please everyone. Do you put your needs or wants after your husband's or boyfriend's and your children's?

Years ago women seldom worked away from home. They were expected to take care of the children and have food on the table at mealtimes. They may have eaten only after everyone else was served. They were considered as almost second-class citizens. Men were the important people in the world. That is where the "pleaser" idea came from—the role that women were expected to fill.

Today women's roles have changed. Women are doctors, pilots, lawyers, and leaders in business and government. They work as secretaries, nurses, teachers, and store clerks, but also as electricians, construction workers, and telephone installers. It no longer makes sense for women to spend long hours at work and yet be expected to please everyone at home, too.

As a woman, you have a right to be your own person. Family life should be everybody's job, not just yours. Your mate does not have the right to hit you if dinner is not on the table when expected or to think that housework and child care are "women's work." Do not continue to do everything yourself and feel angry inside. Speak up; you will never get help if you do not ask for it.

Of course, if you have small children there are things you *must* do to care for them. They are unable to take care of themselves and depend on you to do it. While they are small, you can *never* leave them unsupervised, even for just a few minutes. You will have little time for yourself, and there will be days when you are totally "fed up" with taking care of children. As soon as they are older, try to teach them to do things for themselves so that they will learn that mothers have rights, too.

What things do you do to please others? . . . Are you easily talked into going places and doing things because other people want to— even though you would rather not? . . . If someone gives you a few cents less than the right change at a store, do you ask for what you did not get? . . . If you try on several pairs of shoes at a store, do you feel you have to buy at least one pair? . . . Do you jump up to wait on your mate or children whenever they want something? . . . Does your family know how to make you feel guilty? . . . These are the kinds of things you can change. You can learn to be assertive and tell other people what *you* want and need and not continue to live your life as a second-class citizen.

• How do you treat others? Do you like the way others treat you? Do you listen when people talk and really *care* about them? Can they tell you care by the way you act? Do you get mad without much reason and say things you feel bad about later? Do you start arguments, or do you try to stop them? Do you tell people, "That is just the way I am," as an excuse for not trying to change? Think about all those questions and what your answers are.

Can you change? What do you think? It is no accident how we get along with other people; we *choose* what we say and do, and we can *choose* to do it differently. How do you react when you have problems? Do you see them as ways to grow and learn from them, or do you give up? Do you try to lose yourself in drugs or alcohol or even by staying out late or overworking? Those actions do not *solve* problems, even though you may feel better for a little while. In the end, they may even create *more* problems. Everyone has problems; they are a part of life. You cannot escape, but you can decide to fight back instead of giving up. It is not the *problem* that causes you trouble, it is how you handle it. You can choose to take your problems out on someone else by arguing or hitting someone, or even with a gun. Or you can reason with people; tell them what you want or need, and try to settle your arguments peacefully.

If this is hard for you, tell yourself you want to get along better with just *one* person. Keep telling yourself what you want to do and *choose* how you are going to act toward that one person. If you *act* differently, they will have to *react* differently. You do not have the power to change *them*, but you do have the power to change *you*. Life does not have to just "happen" to you. (Time: 5 minutes.)

• Ask participants to turn to the "Passive," "Assertive," and "Aggressive" pages in their handbooks. Ask if anyone can explain what each of those terms means. The facilitator should now read aloud the pages in the handbook. (Time: 25 minutes.)

PASSIVE BEHAVIOR

If you behave passively, you do not say what you really mean or tell people how you feel. You let others take advantage of you. You do what you are told, even if inside you do not really want to. You may feel mad at others or yourself. You may cry or only hint at what you want and expect others to read your mind. If you try to please everyone else, avoid fighting or arguing, or give in so people will like you, you are being passive.

When You Act Passively, You:

Never say what you really want; others have to guess what it is

Say "I'm sorry" and "I guess" too much

Let other people tell you what to do and how you feel

Do not speak up for yourself

May feel tense or shaky

Look down and do not look others in the eye

Walk like a victim, not a powerful person

AGGRESSIVE BEHAVIOR

If you are aggressive, you tell others how you really think or feel about something, but you make other people angry because of your attitude. You blame and threaten them, point or shake your finger at them, yell insults, and demand what you want *now*. You may even fight to get your own way. Maybe you *will* get what you want, but you will not feel good about it, and neither will others.

When You Act Aggressively, You:

Blame others with "you" statements
Look angry, threaten others, or shake your finger at them
Are usually loud, may yell, and insist on what you want "right now"
Accuse others and tell them what they "need" to do

"You" Statements Blame Others:

You made me——; You always——; You never——; You charged me too much——; You got my order wrong——.

ASSERTIVE BEHAVIOR

If you are an assertive person, you express your true thoughts and feelings in ways that do not hurt others. You say what you really want or need and are willing to stand up for yourself, but you do not run over people to do so. You think about what other people need and want, too, and try to work things out without making them mad. You feel relaxed and good about yourself.

When You Act Assertively, You:

Use "I" statements
Say what you really want, feel, or think
Do not say things to hurt other people
Are reasonable
Listen to the other person
Use a pleasant voice and look at them

"I" Messages Tell Others How You Feel:

I feel angry when you—; I get upset when—; I think
   you may have made a mistake—; I have been wait-
ing
   a long time—.

IF YOU ARE PASSIVE, YOU FEEL:

Hurt, unhappy, and mad at yourself.

IF YOU ARE AGGRESSIVE, YOU FEEL:

Better than others, "right," angry, on edge, as if others are trying to take advantage of you.

IF YOU ARE ASSERTIVE, YOU FEEL:

Relaxed, honest, as if you deserve respect, in charge of your life.

WHEN YOU ARE PASSIVE, OTHERS FEEL:

Angry with you because they are not sure what you want, better than you are.

WHEN YOU ARE AGGRESSIVE, OTHERS FEEL:

Hurt, angry, as if they have to protect themselves from your attack, insulted or "put down."

WHEN YOU ARE ASSERTIVE, OTHERS FEEL:

That you are being reasonable, that you understand their point of view, that you can work out an agreement.

IF YOU ARE PASSIVE:

You want everyone to like you.
You want to please everyone.

But Instead:

You hardly ever get what you want.
Other people take advantage of you.
You feel angry inside but are afraid to show it outside.
You may take that anger out on others.
You may have headaches or other physical symptoms.
You feel lonely and isolated.

IF YOU ARE AGGRESSIVE:

You want to be in power.
You want to put others down.
You want to frighten others into doing what you want.

But Instead:

You may get what you want, but you have to hurt others to get it.
People want to "get even" with you.
You do not respect the rights of others.
You feel "uptight."
Others do not like or respect you.

IF YOU ARE ASSERTIVE:

You want to express your true feelings, wants, and
   needs.
You respect others and want them to respect you.

And What Happens Is:

You usually get what you want, if it is within reason.
You feel good about yourself.
You respect the rights of others.
You can work out an agreement that is good for both
   sides.

ROLE-PLAYS:
WHAT DO YOU DO?

Role-play #1: You are in a restaurant and the service is terrible. You had to wait almost an hour for your food, and it is cold when you get it. How do you handle it?

- If you are passive? . . . (Do not say anything, and maybe do not leave a tip so they will know you were unhappy.)
- If you are aggressive? . . . (Scream at the waitress, tell her what you think of her and the service, and cause a scene.)
- If you are assertive? . . . (Calmly tell the cashier when you leave that you were very displeased with the service and explain why, and maybe they will make an adjustment in your bill.)

Role-play #2: You are at a resource agency office. They tell you the paperwork you brought is not complete. You have to complete it before they can see you, so today's appointment is canceled. How do you handle it?

- If you are passive? . . . (You hang your head and leave without trying to explain why.)
- If you are aggressive? . . . (You scream, make a scene, threaten the worker.)
- If you are assertive? . . . (You explain that you have applied for the needed document, but it is not back yet. Ask if you can see the worker to tell her that.)

Role-play #3: Your friend calls on the phone and tells you about a problem she has been having. You have to leave to pick up your children at school. How do you handle it?

- If you are passive? . . . (You keep listening, while you get more and more upset about being late to pick up your children; you finally make up an excuse to get off the phone.)
- If you are aggressive? . . . (You say, "Why do you always have to dump on me? I have things to do, and I am too busy to listen to you.")

- If you are assertive? . . . (You say, "I have to go pick up the children at school, but call me back in thirty minutes, and we can talk then.")

- Anger is a scary emotion. You may feel that it is not okay to be angry, or that if you let your anger out, you will not be able to control it, and you may do something terrible. Maybe you heard your parents argue, or maybe they had physical fights that you could not stop. You might think that if you become angry, people will not like you or that you do not have a right to get mad. The things you fear will happen if you get angry are more likely to happen if you do not *allow* yourself to get angry. What happens when you try not to get angry? How do you feel? . . . (headaches, upset stomach, anxiety, heart pounding, depression, take it out on others) If you keep the anger inside, it is like a balloon that is blown up bigger and bigger until it bursts. If you let out a little of the anger once in a while, you will not have to worry about the balloon bursting when things get really bad. You will not say those angry words you cannot take back.

Maybe your parents never let you be angry at them or anybody else. They could yell at you, but you could not yell back. Or they may have buried their anger with alcohol, drugs, or depression. You can bury anger under lots of behaviors—overeating, trying to please everyone but yourself, having sex with lots of people, or even getting sick.

You may have the opposite problem from burying your anger, you may be angry all the time, yelling and screaming and becoming someone nobody wants to be around.

Some ways to manage your anger better are:

- Give yourself permission to be angry. It is a normal feeling, such as being happy or sad. You are not *bad* if you are angry, or good, or right, or wrong.
- Do something with your anger. Hit a pillow, or go somewhere by yourself and yell out loud. Clean house. Go for a walk. Tell somebody you trust how mad you are. Do *not* hit someone! Take a deep breath, count to ten, and leave the area. Violence

does not solve anything. It is better to walk away than be carried away.

The way you act may not always please those around you. Do you constantly complain about things, even things that cannot be changed, such as traffic, weather, long waits, being sick, or not being listened to? . . . Do you know someone like that? . . . Complaining makes you feel bad, makes you angry and frustrated, and attracts other people who complain about everything, too. Soon you can no longer see the positives in life. Try to change the way you see things. Instead of complaining about the weather, use a rainy day to read a book or try a new receipe. Instead of complaining about your long wait to see the doctor, be glad there is a doctor you can see, even though you have to wait. Complaining saps energy you could use to solve a problem or make a choice. Be a happy, positive person—one other people want to be around. (Time: 15 minutes.)

• Distribute evaluation forms; have pencils available. Names are optional. Collect them facedown on one of the tables. (Time: 5 minutes.)

• Hold the Pretty Prize drawing. Be sure all group members are entered. The same person cannot win two weeks in succession. (Time: 5 minutes.)

• Do the Car Wash exercise if time permits.

Chapter 6

Week Four: My Appearance

Goals for the Week Are:

1. To find out what participants like and dislike about their bodies
2. To discuss basic hygiene, clean body, hair, and clothing
3. To have a speaker, if possible, who can teach the participants beauty-related subjects. These could include basic makeup, skin care, haircuts and care, flattering colors and clothing.
4. To increase self-esteem through improved appearance

Materials Needed:

A Participant Handbook for each group member
Pens, felt-tip markers, and paper or notebook for sign-in
Name tags
Pencils for participants
Assorted colors of construction paper for small hearts for each group member (about three inches across). "I'm perfect inside" should be printed in the middle of each heart.
Pins or tape, so hearts can be worn by participants during the session
Combs or basic beauty items can be distributed, if desired
Chalkboard, flip chart, or large pad of drawing paper
Pretty Prize(s)

Improved appearance is the focus of this week. Looking better results in feeling better about yourself. Many persons going through the LAMS program have little self-esteem, and it often shows in their appearance.

Begin this week's session by having all group members turn to the Affirmation for Week Four in their handbooks. Read it aloud, in unison.

Before the session, cut out small paper hearts with "I'm perfect inside" printed on them. Give each participant one, along with a pin or tape, so they can wear it during the session. How you look is important to how you feel, and the activities for this session point this out. Discuss general appearance, best and worst features, favorite colors, hairstyles, and basic hygiene.

Some group members may have dirty, uncombed, or poorly cut hair. Their makeup may be nonexistent or overdone. Their clothing may be dirty, stained, or ill-fitting, with no attempts made to repair clothing that is torn or has ripped seams. They may have unbrushed teeth or body odor. Those are often indicators of depression or a feeling that nobody cares how they look, least of all themselves. There is almost always an improvement in appearance over the course of participation in LAMS. Part of this may be because of the content of the program, but it is also the result of peer pressure from the group and the participant's own feelings of improved self-worth.

Basic good hygiene can be addressed by the leader, but having a speaker is also helpful. There are many possibilities. Beauticians, beauty company representatives, hairdressers, beauty school teachers, or home economics teachers are a few choices. If a speaker cannot be located, there are many books in the library on such subjects, and the facilitator can prepare the program. There are also some videos that can be used. Makeovers can be done during the group, but care needs to be taken that the other members do not get restless or bored. Color charts for skin tones and haircolor are helpful in choosing flattering clothing, and every participant can be analyzed during the session and given suggestions. The videos listed in the resources section at the back of this book can be used as springboards for discussion, but the group often becomes bored if that is the entire program. Using parts of them has proven to be more effective. If male participants make up part of the LAMS group, they can also benefit from learning to choose their best clothing colors and the importance of basic hygiene and good grooming.

The speaker can continue both before and after the break and mealtime. More than one speaker could be invited to speak on different topics.

Conclude the session as always with evaluations, the Pretty Prize drawing, and the Car Wash exercise. Since this session highlights appearance, an extra Pretty Prize could be given, or beauty product samples might be distributed to all the group members.

WEEK FOUR: MY APPEARANCE

• After registration, all new members get a Participant Handbook and Pre-LAMS Questionnaire to be completed and handed in at the end of the session.

• Introduce facilitator(s) and briefly describe the LAMS program and discuss houskeeping issues. (Time: 5 minutes.)

• Read the Affirmation aloud, in unison; participants should read from their handbooks. (Time: 5 minutes.)

> I choose to look good, to be clean and well-groomed,
>   not just for others, but for myself.
> I will keep my clothing washed and in good repair,
>   even if that is sometimes hard to do.
> I will learn as much as I can about how I can improve
>   my appearance.
> I will practice what I learn with my family.

• Pass out the premade paper hearts to each group member and have them wear the hearts during the session.

• Hold a discussion about appearance. Ask all group members the following questions (Time: 20 minutes):

> What are you best features? What part of your body is
> your favorite and most attractive? . . . What is your least

favorite feature? . . . What is your favorite color? . . . Do you think it looks good on you when you wear it? . . . Do other people tell you that you look your best when wearing that color? . . . What about your hair? Do you like it long or short, curly or straight? . . . Which looks best on you, and why do you like it? . . . Do you ever wear makeup? . . . Why or why not? . . . (If you wish to distribute a comb or beauty item, do it now.)

Basic hygiene consists of keeping your body, your hair, and your clothing clean. Bathing often, brushing your teeth regularly, and using deodorant are all necessary if you want to feel good about yourself. You may not recognize bad breath or body odor, but others around you will. If your hair is not washed often, it will look dull and oily and will be hard to manage. Clothing can be kept clean and in good repair, whether expensive or from Goodwill. You can choose clothing that fits well and is flattering and is neither too tight nor too loose. If you have children, be sure they follow good hygiene habits, also, so others will want to be around them.

Part of caring for your body is eating properly, not eating all junk foods. Weight control and fitness are other concerns. Exercise makes you feel better and look better and can help to reduce your weight, if necessary, and relieve stress. It can be as simple as taking a daily walk or as involved as a regular exercise routine.

• Introduce the guest speaker. This person may be a beautician or cosmetologist who speaks on hair and skin care, colors, makeup, clothing, or any subject related to appearance. If necessary, two different speakers may come; have another scheduled for after the break. They may be recruited from local beauty schools, department stores, the Department of Agriculture, beauty consultants, etc.

If a speaker cannot be located, the facilitator can visit the local library and find books on many beauty-related subjects and make their own presentation. Current magazines also could be a good source of information or material that could be copied and handed out to group members. There are also videos available on makeup and colors that could replace or enhance a speaker's presentation. Two possibilities are, *Hot Makeup, Tips for That Cool Look,* Simitar Entertainment, Inc., Minnesota; and *Color and You,* Clare Revelli (1987), Simon and Schuster Video. (Time: 30 minutes.)

• Announce time for a break and food. Children may eat with adults if desired. (Time: 30 minutes.)

• Continue with a speaker after break. Possible activities are makeup or hairstyles tried on volunteers, color charts, figure types, and clothing selection. "Before" and "After" pictures are fun. (Time: 45 minutes.)

• Distribute evaluation forms; have pencils available. Names are optional. Collect them facedown on one of the tables. (Time: 5 minutes.)

• Hold the Pretty Prize drawing. Since the session today has focused on appearance, you may want to award an extra Pretty Prize. (Time: 5 minutes.)

• Do the Car Wash self-esteem exercise if time allows. (Time: 5 minutes.)

Chapter 7

Week Five: My Time for Myself

Goals for the Week Are:

1. To learn that everyone deserves time for themselves
2. To learn to express feelings to music
3. To try a craft activity so they realize that they can make something pretty or useful

Materials Needed:

A Participant Handbook for each group member
Pens, felt-tip markers, and paper or notebook for sign-in
Name tags
Pencils for participants
Cassette player
Cassette of music chosen for the "Expressing Yourself" exercise
Colored chalks or nonoil pastels or watercolors and brushes
Varied colors of 12″ × 18″ construction paper
Wet paper towels for cleanup
Hairspray to set chalk drawings, if desired
Necessary materials for selected craft project
Chalkboard, flip chart, or large pad of drawing paper
Pretty Prize(s)

Many participants in the LAMS program have never even considered taking time for themselves or felt that they deserved to do so. Begin this week's session with the usual routine. Then ask participants to turn to Week Five in their handbooks and read the Affirmation aloud, in unison. Then the leader should read "Just Be You," with group members following along in their handbooks.

Most LAMS members have never had an opportunity to express their feelings to music or to notice that music *creates* feelings. The second activity, "Expressing Yourself to Music," helps them recognize and illustrate how music makes them *feel*. They do not have to draw anything recognizable, though they can if they wish; they just use colors to express the mood of the music. There has been only one complaint about this activity over the five years it has been used in this program—a member said this was childish and refused to draw at all. The facilitator should select a piece of music that has a clear mood, preferably without words, as they can be distracting. Listen to the music in advance of the session and possibly create a sample picture of what you want. After you have repeated this session several times, you will have examples from past group members. Participants can keep their creations, hand them in for use as future examples, or throw them away. This is a very messy activity; before the craft project is attempted, wet paper towels should be provided to clean up hands and tables when the exercise is over.

Most of the time for this session is spent on crafts. Gather needed materials prior to the session, as it can prove hectic if you are not well-prepared in advance. If possible, have the break and meal before beginning so the tables will be cleaned off for the rest of the session. Very few group members will have attempted a craft project in the past, and many have never succeeded in completing anything in their lives. They are empowered by the idea that they can successfully create something beautiful or useful. They begin the project feeling inadequate but finish with satisfaction.

Any craft can be attempted, as long it is fairly simple and the materials do not cost too much. Hair bows, especially, are very economical for women to make yet are quite expensive to buy. If the group includes men, beaded key rings are a good project. Both can be made for either adults or children and are easy enough that everyone should have something to be proud of when the project is completed. Some group members may need help at first, but all will be more confident by the end of the session. Explain the cost of materials used and how practice could result in possibly salable items and certainly in gifts.

Special craft projects are often included in regular sessions near major holidays: baskets and spoon bunnies at Easter; potpourri sachets at Valentine's Day; angels at Christmas. Any nearby craft store or holiday magazine should have many possibilities along with directions. Budgetary restrictions and time constraints will be the major concerns. Be sure that any craft attempted is not too difficult. You are trying to build successes, not failures.

End the session with evaluations, the Pretty Prize drawing, and the Car Wash exercise, if there is time. This week's activities often run overtime, as everyone rushes to complete their projects.

WEEK FIVE: MY TIME FOR MYSELF

• After registration, all new members get a Participant Handbook and Pre-LAMS Questionnaire to be completed and handed in at the end of the session. Facilitators may wish to place assorted chalks and wet paper towels for each group member on the tables before the session begins to save time later on.

• Introduce facilitator(s) and briefly describe the LAMS program and discuss housekeeping issues. (Time: 5 minutes.)

• Read the Affirmation aloud, in unison; participants should read from their handbooks. (Time: 5 minutes.)

> I can allow myself to be different from everyone else and
>   still be okay.
> I can have feelings and be warm and kind.
> I can allow myself to like me as I am.
> I can do "fun" things because I want to, without a reason.
> I will allow myself to do what *I* want to do, just for *me*,
>   because I deserve it.
> I will make time every day to do at least one nice thing
>   for myself, not always for others.
> Allowing myself to be happy makes me feel better
>   about myself.

• The facilitator should read aloud, "Just Be You." Participants should follow along in their handbooks. (Time: 5 minutes.)

JUST BE YOU

"It is okay to be different. You do not have to be just like your mother, or your father, or anyone else in your family. You do not have to be what other people want you to be; you can just be you. Being different is what makes other people want to know you and like you.

Can you imagine how dull it would be if everyone were just alike? Everyone would have the same color hair and eyes and would look the same. When a baby was born, nobody would have to wonder what it would look like; they would already know. All the houses and cars would look alike; even all of the business buildings would look alike because everyone would like the same things. Nobody would be tall or short, or fat or thin. Nobody would be sad or happy, or funny or grouchy. That would be a terrible world.

It is all right to make mistakes or to forget things. That is part of being human, and no humans are perfect. It is better to make a mistake than not to try at all. You can change your mind if you want to and change your whole life if you choose to. You can take time every day to do something for yourself, not always for others. You can take time to be happy, to laugh, to sing, and to enjoy being alive.

Learn to enjoy just being *you*!

• The "Expressing Yourself to Music" exercise is based on an exercise in *Action Speaks Louder,* by Remocker and Storch (pp. 113-114). Music chosen should be instrumental; classical is best because it usually does not have lyrics, which could influence feelings. Some possibilities are: "Moonlight Sonata," by Beethoven; "Ave Maria," by Schubert; "Nutcracker Suite," by Tchaikovsky; "William Tell Overture," by Rossini; and "Adagio for Trumpet and Organ," by Albinoni. Any music selected should last three to five minutes and spark imaginations or evoke feelings through tempo or instruments. Make sure all participants have chalks or paints and wet paper towels for cleanup. Give each participant a sheet of 12-by-18-inch construction paper, in any color desired. Have the musical selection ready to play on a cassette or CD player. Explain the exercise as follows (Time: 20 minutes):

EXPRESSING YOURSELF TO MUSIC

This exercise helps express feelings. You may have done something like this when you were in school, or you may never have done it before. I am going to play a piece of music through twice. The first time just listen to it quietly and try to be aware of how it makes you feel. The second time, while it is playing, try to put those feelings down on your paper. You can use any colors, and you do not have to draw a picture of anything, though you can if you want to. You may want to use color to express happiness or sadness, or maybe you will use curved or straight lines. The music may sound like anger, or waves, or running water, or mountains. When you finish, you may want to tell the rest of us why you put down what you did, but you do not have to. This picture is for you; it does not have to be turned in.

Play the music through once. Then tell everyone to get ready to draw when it starts again. The leader may want to draw, also. When the music concludes, turn if off, but let anyone finish who has not done so. Ask if anyone wants to describe his or her picture. Hairspray can be used as a fixative for the chalk, if desired.

• Introduce the craft activity. Making hair bows is a craft that is inexpensive and easy to master, and everyone can make something useful and pretty. Any other simple craft fitting into the allotted time could be used. If a holiday is near, a special project could be completed with that theme. Men can make beaded keyrings at the same time women are making hair bows, if it is a mixed group. Break time may need to be held earlier so craft materials are not on the tables when the meal is eaten. (Time: 25 minutes.)

• Announce time for a break and food. Children may eat with adults if desired. (Time: 30 minutes.)

• Begin the craft, which can be anything that fits the time period and has a high probability of success. Bow-making is a good choice for women. (Time: 50 minutes.)

Supplies needed:

> *Any type ribbon.* The stiffer types, sometimes as little as 10¢ per yard, are easier to work with but crush more easily. Widths of more than one and one-half inches are difficult. The most durable is grosgrain ribbon, but it is the most expensive.
>
> *Hot glue guns,* regular or low-melt. Low-melt guns are safer, as the glue does not burn when touched. These can be found for $1.99 to $3.99 in most cases.
>
> *Glue sticks,* about 10¢ to 25¢ cents each.
>
> *Barrette backs,* available at craft stores for as little as 9¢ each.
>
> *Fine craft wire,* can be flower wire, copper, or fine steel. It costs about $3.00 for a large spool, which is enough for hundreds of bows.
>
> *Scissors,* several pairs, ideally a pair for each participant.
>
> *Measuring tape,* one or two for the leaders to measure ribbon and wire; precutting both saves time.
>
> *Instruction book.* A simple, very good one is "Hair Bows for Kids," by Gick Publishing, Inc., 1990. You can find this is in craft stores. It has clear photographs of many different types of bows and how to make them.

Most ribbons need to be cut into one-yard pieces, with a few shorter pieces for baby-bows and longer ones (up to two yards) for the largest barrettes. Different widths and types of ribbon, as well as lace and even colored shoe laces, can be used. They can be combined and overlaid as desired. Wire needs to be cut in 12- to 36-inch lengths, depending on the type of bow. Loop-type bows are the simplest; succeeding loops are wired to the barrette back; double or triple bows of the regular type are hot-glued to the barrette back. Leaders will probably want to get a book and practice first before attempting to teach the skill to others. Someone who is proficient at bow-making could be asked to instruct the group if preferred.

This craft is easily mastered, and participants can make something both attractive and useful. It is a good self-esteem builder, as many group members have never attempted craft projects, and are surprised they can succeed. Some participants have bought their own materials and made more bows for their family or to sell. Another advantage of this craft is that the necessary materials are relatively inexpensive. If there are men in the group, the leaders should use a different craft, such as making beaded keyrings.

In addition to this craft session, a short project may be included in any session preceding a holiday. Possible craft ideas are drawer sachets with potpourri inside lace or net squares, tied with ribbon, for both Christmas and Valentine's Day and small grapevine wreaths decorated with ribbons and beads for Christmas. Easter baskets can be made from small plastic bowls by attaching chenille handles and filling them with cellophane grass and candy. Craft books and magazines have numerous ideas for every holiday. Try them yourself first; remember that a project which is too hard to master does little for anyone's self-esteem.

• Distribute evaluation forms; have pencils available. Names are optional. Collect them facedown on one of the tables. (Time: 5 minutes.)

• Hold the Pretty Prize drawing. Be sure all group members are entered. The same person cannot win two weeks in succession. (Time: 5 minutes.)

• Do the Car Wash exercise if there is time; this is usually a hard session to end, as members are trying to finish their projects.

Chapter 8

Week Six: My Friends

Goals for the Week Are:

1. To learn what a good friend is and is not
2. To learn how friends influence your life
3. To learn other group member's feelings through the "Ungame"

Materials Needed:

A Participant Handbook for each group member
Pens, felt-tip markers, and paper or notebook for sign-in
Name tags
Pencils for participants
Sheets of paper for writing attributes of a good friend
The "Ungame" or similar activity or exercise
Chalkboard, flip chart, or large pad of drawing paper
Pretty Prize(s)

How to make friends, how to be a good friend, and the good or bad influence of friends are the main lessons to be taught this week. Many participants in the LAMS program have problems choosing friends and are continually drawn into bad situations because they make poor choices.

After the usual settling down, introductions, and any announcements, have all group members open their handbooks to Week Six and read the Affirmation aloud, in unison. Then, the facilitator should read "Putty People" aloud, while participants follow along in their handbooks. Discuss whether participants allow others to shape them as others would prefer them to be.

The game, "Gossip," is the first activity. All should be familiar with this from childhood. The facilitator should whisper a bit of juicy gossip about a fictional person or family to the first person on their right. Each succeeding person whispers what they heard to the next, on around the group. The last person tells the group what they heard, and the beginning facilitator reads what she *really* said. There are usually tremendous differences between the two, and it can then be explained that gossip works exactly that way. Group members need to remember that gossip they hear, whether from friends or strangers, may have little resemblance to the truth. It also shows that what is said behind one's back is not necessarily the truth.

"Blind Run" is an optional activity but can be a useful illustration of trust. Some group members are quite uncomfortable doing this and may refuse to participate. Because of such protests, the "Gossip" game is usually the one used.

Next, have LAMS members pair up and write down qualities they want their friends to have. After a few minutes, ask them to volunteer aloud some of the things they have written and write them on the chalkboard or flip chart. Ask if they have those qualities themselves.

That activity leads into "How to be a Friend," which is in the group members' handbooks. Ask them to turn to that reading in Week Six. Some participants may know how they want their friends to be but may not realize how to make and keep friends themselves. They may always choose the wrong men or women for intimate relationships or again become involved in drug or criminal activities because of association with friends who continue those pursuits. They may try to be an "only" friend to someone, smothering them with their constant presence and not letting them see anyone else. They may take advantage of their friends, then wonder at their cool reception when they ask for a favor. There are many opportunities for interaction in the group and discussions of what makes a good friend and what are the best and worst things a friend has ever done.

Finally, the "Ungame" or another similar activity helps the group become aware of how other people feel or react in certain situations, so they realize that everyone is different, and those differences are to be appreciated. These questions have proven very popular, as most participants enjoy sharing their thoughts and feelings with others in the group and sometimes comment on answers given by others. You will probably not finish all of the questions; ask them around the group, including the leaders, as time permits. Then, go on to the closing evaluations, the Pretty Prize drawing, and the Car Wash exercise.

WEEK SIX: MY FRIENDS

• Register all new members and give each a Participant Handbook and Pre-Lams Questionnaire to be completed and handed in at the end of the session.

• Introduce facilitator(s) and briefly describe the LAMS program and discuss housekeeping issues. (Time: 5 minutes.)

• Read the Affirmation aloud, in unison; participants should read from their handbooks. (Time: 5 minutes.)

> I will learn to love myself.
> I am a worthwhile person.
> I deserve to be happy.
> I do not have to please everyone.
> I deserve to be loved and respected by others.
> I will choose friends that make me feel good about myself.

• Read "Putty People" aloud; participants should follow along in their handbooks. Discuss afterward. (Time: 10 minutes.)

PUTTY PEOPLE

Are you a "putty person," one who shapes yourself exactly as someone else wants you to? Do you want so much to be liked that you give up what *you* want for what *others* want? Do you pretend you have no likes or dislikes of your own, no opinions of your own, and bend yourself all out of shape to be the person someone else wants you to be?

Putty people never make their own decisions; they wait for someone else to tell them what to decide. They never tell anyone else where they want to eat, what movie they want to see, or what they want to do on the weekend.

The worst thing about being a putty person is that you change yourself into the shape someone else wants you to be, and you forget what you looked like to begin with. Pretty soon you are no longer yourself at all; you are squeezed into a new and different shape, and you have no memory of what you used to be.

Do not let others make you a putty person; stand up for yourself; express yourself; and be the kind of special person that makes other people want *your* opinion.

• Initiate a game, either "Gossip" or "Blind Run." "Blind Run" is based on a game in *Action Speaks Louder*, by Remocker and Storch (p. 154). (Time: 10 minutes.)

GOSSIP

This is an old game that you may have played as children. It is about discovering who your friends really are—whether you can believe what they say at first, or whether they speak differently behind your back.

Ask participants to sit or stand in a circle. Designate a first person and a last person. Whisper in the ear of the first person two or three sentences of some type of juicy but fictional gossip. (Something such as, "I heard that Mary caught her husband Don kissing her best friend in their apartment when she came home from taking the kids to a movie. She threw them both out and plans to get a divorce.")

They repeat what they think you said to the next person, and so on, around to the last member. Ask both the first and last person to repeat what they heard, and then tell them what the original message was. This illustrates what happens to facts when they are repeated over and over; they soon have little resemblance to the truth.

BLIND RUN

This is an optional activity; you need to have a large enough open space.

Have the group members form an oval, with everyone standing about two feet apart. Ask someone to volunteer to be in the middle. Blindfold the volunteer or shut his or her eyes, and then turn the person around three or four times until the person loses the sense of direction. The volunteer then walks rapidly forward until stopped, turned around, and redirected across the oval. This continues until the volunteer says he or she is ready to stop. The person in the middle has to trust the other group members for redirection and not allow him or her to be hurt. Next, ask for another volunteer, or select someone, until everyone has had a chance to be in the center.

The objective of this exercise is to build trust through having to depend on others and having others depend on you. Trust is a part of most friendships.

• Have the group members count off into pairs and decide what qualities make a good friend. Pass out one sheet of paper to each group of two. Each pair is to decide what qualities make a good friend, and one member writes down the suggestions. After a few minutes, have them stop. Ask participants to call out the qualities they feel are important, and write them on the chalkboard or a large pad of paper. Discuss why these are the qualities they look for in a friend, and ask if they see the same qualities in themselves. (Time: 15 minutes.)

• Have group members turn in their handbooks to "How To Be a Friend." (Time: 20 minutes.)

HOW TO BE A FRIEND

Show respect and consideration for others.

If other people always take advantage of you, ask yourself how you are acting to make them treat you that way. Maybe *you* have to change.

Do not scream at people to make them do what you want; it does not work.

Tell other people when they do a good job, and tell them why you believe in them.

You do not have to agree with everything someone says to be his or her friend. Differences make people more interesting.

Ask questions before you accept gossip; what you heard may not be true.

Do not tell people things for "their own good." This often hurts feelings.

Do not complain about your life or about things you cannot control.

Be dependable; do what you say you will do.

Do not be afraid to admit you are wrong.

Do not be afraid to care about others; be there for them, or listen to them.

Get other people's opinions, but make up your own mind. You do not need permission to live your own life.

Be an example; do not just tell others what to do.

Reach out to meet new people; do not always wait for them to make the first move.

True friends are not made overnight. Anyone who wants to be your best friend immediately may have something else in mind.

Remember, only *you* can make yourself happy; nobody else can do it for you.

People usually do not give a lot of thought to what they want from their friends. Why do you consider someone your friend? Is she helpful, caring, dependable, and always there when you are down? Can you have the same relationship with everyone—your boss, your doctor, or the cashier at the grocery store? Probably you cannot; all of our friendships are different because we want different things from different people.

Do not expect your friends to be perfect. They may let you down, just as you may let them down sometimes. They may have had a bad day or said something that hurt your feelings without meaning to. Expect the best, but do not give up on them if they fall short once in a while. Talk it out; do not go away mad.

What you want out of a friendship may not be the same as what your friend wants. Find out what she wants from you, as well as what you want from her. Do not expect your friends to be with you every minute, and especially—do not expect her to be your *only* friend. Being jealous of her time and attention can break up your friendship. You need other friends just as she does.

It is great to have friends to share your troubles, your joys, and just to talk with. But there are limits. Do you say hurtful things and insult them? Just because someone is your friend does not give you the right to tell her all of her faults, tell her she looks terrible, or hurt her in any way. Saying that you did not mean it does not make her feel better.

Do you take advantage of your friends, always taking from them and never giving to them? Most people do not mind helping you out sometimes, but if you want a friend to take you to the grocery store one day, downtown the next, and to a doctor appointment the next, she may begin to feel you only want her for a friend because she has a car.

Do you ask a friend to take care of your children for "just a little while" and not come back for hours? Do that several times, and your friend will refuse to help you at all. Do you borrow from her constantly, so that she says to herself, "Oh, no . . . here she comes again!" when she sees you coming to the door?

In order to have friends you must realize that they have lives, too. Treat them the way you would like to be treated.

Discuss the above suggestions for making and keeping friends.

• Announce time for a break and food. Children may eat with adults if desired. (Time: 30 minutes.)

• Do you lead a very isolated, lonely life? You can live in a crowded house and still feel lonely. Loneliness is one of the most common problems people face. Women tend to be alone with their children much of the time. Have you ever wished you could talk to someone over the age of three or four? . . . Conversation with small children usually consists of a long string of orders or no-no's. Those are necessary, but they do not do a lot for your need to talk to and share ideas with another person. Men sometimes do not understand why women meet them at the door when they arrive home, wanting to share all the day's happenings, bad or good, before they have time to sit down and catch their breath. The reason is that women have had nobody to really "talk to" all day, while their mates have talked so much they want to be quiet for a while.

Have you ever been stuck at home for several days or weeks because your children, one after the other, caught some contagious ailment and you could not leave the house? . . . Talk about "cabin fever!" I am sure the early settlers of this country had even worse problems, such as being snowed in or having their nearest neighbors twenty miles away before the days of automobiles. No wonder the few neighborhood social activities were so well attended.

Let's conduct a check on your own need for friendships and how you fulfill that need. Do you feel sometimes that nobody really cares about you or what you think or feel? . . . Do you have trouble knowing what to do or say to make friends? . . . Do you have someone you can share your feelings with—a friend, relative, or your mate? . . . Does not having someone leave you feeling empty and as if there is something missing in your life? . . . If so, you need to make some friends, reach out and be a friend to someone else, or join a group or organization to meet some other people. Do you attend a church? That is a good place to meet people with similar ideas and feelings, and they always have social activities as well as religious services. Your local library has many programs that can involve both you and your children. You can even study there for your GED (general equivalency diploma, which is similar to a high school diploma) if you do not have one. If you live in a housing project or an apartment, you may have special activities with other residents. Your neighborhood community or recreation centers have regularly scheduled programs, also. Can any of you think of other places where you can or have made friends? . . . (Time: 20 minutes.)

• What is the best thing a friend has ever done for you? . . . What is the worst experience you have ever had with someone you thought was your friend? . . . (Time: 10 minutes.)

• Play the "Ungame." This is a game that is available at many large toy stores or by mail order from retailers of counseling or educational materials. It comes with a game board, but the board is difficult to use with a large group. Instead, try using just the question cards, asking them one by one around the group, with each person answering succeeding questions. These are good discussion starters, which help the group members get acquainted with each other and discover how they really feel about themselves, their friends, and family. Sample questions are: "Complete the sentence: The person who has influenced me the most in my life is _____." or "How do you respond when someone criticizes you?" or "To whom can you turn if you need to be comforted?" (Time: 20 minutes.)

Another activity could be used here if you are unable to find the "Ungame."

• Distribute evaluation forms; have pencils available. Names are optional. Collect them facedown on one of the tables. (Time: 5 minutes.)

• Hold the Pretty Prize drawing. Be sure all group members are entered. The same person cannot win two weeks in succession. (Time: 5 minutes.)

• Do the Car Wash exercise if time allows.

Chapter 9

Week Seven: My Education

Goals for the Week Are:

1. To learn why everyone needs an education
2. To learn how to get more education or job training
3. To learn how to set a job goal and how to achieve that goal
4. To have a speaker who can present information on local opportunities

Materials Needed:

A Participant Handbook for each group member
Pens, felt-tip markers, and paper or notebook for sign-in
Name tags
Pencils for participants
Handouts on local educational or job-training organizations
  in your area
Chalkboard, flip chart, or large pad of drawing paper
Pretty Prize(s)

The theme for this week is education. Participants may never have thought about why an education is important. They need to be shown the benefits of at least a high school education in terms of the kinds of jobs they can get and the income they can expect from them. Many have no goals and have never considered setting any.

Begin with the Affirmation; read aloud, in unison. There are several readings this week. The facilitator should read aloud "Money," "In Charge," and "Excuses." Participants should follow along in their handbooks.

Lead in to what the speaker will present by asking general questions about education; discuss the kinds of jobs you have to take if you do not have at least a high school diploma or GED. The questions are included in this week's material. There is an optional exercise following the questions, if there is time. It illustrates what participants would like to be and why.

A junior college or university in your area can usually furnish a speaker who can explain what the requirements are to attend the institution. The speaker can also explain how to get financial aid, which is often a necessity. A high school counselor would also be able to give information on how and where to get a GED or how to enroll in college. If no speaker is available, the facilitator can present the program after doing research to see what is offered in his or her area. If you have job-training organizations in your area, such as the Job Training Partnership Act (JTPA) or other government programs, be sure to contact them. Also, your state employment office is a good resource. Be sure to get specifics as to where contacts can be made and agency telephone numbers to give out during this session. Any handouts or brochures you can obtain will make it easier for group participants to make concrete plans to change their lives for the better.

If there is time after the speaker, read aloud "What Things Can I Do Well?" If there is no more time, refer group members to the reading in their handbooks and ask them to think about what jobs their interests might lead them to pursue. Read aloud "Do You Want a Job?", as it mentions the idea of a "goal job" that may be the end result of much planning and not necessarily the job held before training or education is obtained. Some participants may want instant results and want to begin at the "top."

Getting education or training for a better job is within the reach of almost everyone, if they are willing to take the necessary steps to accomplish that goal. Many people in the LAMS program need help realizing that life is in *their* control; they are not controlled by something "out there."

Finish the session with evaluations, the Pretty Prize drawing, and the Car Wash exercise (if time allows).

WEEK SEVEN: MY EDUCATION

• Register all new members and give each a Participant Handbook and Pre-Lams Questionnaire to be completed and handed in at the end of the session.

• Introduce the facilitator(s). Give a brief description of the LAMS program and housekeeping issues. (Time: 5 minutes.)

• Read the Affirmation aloud, in unison; participants should read from their handbooks. (Time: 5 minutes.)

> I am a worthwhile person.
> I can do anything I want to do.
> I can choose to finish school or get more training to get a job,
>   if that is what I want to do.
> I will live my life for myself, not always just for others.
> I will learn who I am and work to become the best person
>   I can be.

• The facilitator should read aloud to the group "Money," by Ogden Nash, and the "In Charge" and "Excuses" readings. Participants can follow along in their handbooks. (Time: 10 minutes.)

MONEY

> O money, money, money,
>   I am not necessarily one of those
>   who think thee holy.
> But I often stop to wonder
>   How thou canst go out so fast
>   When thou comest in so slowly.

> —Ogden Nash

IN CHARGE

> You are in charge of your life.
> No matter what happens to you,
> there are always many things that you control.

You have to decide what you want,
how badly you want it,
and how you will go about getting it.

Set reasonable goals;
work on those goals one at a time,
and you can make your dreams
become reality.

EXCUSES

I cannot be a success because:
My family was poor.
I have little education.
I have physical limitations.
I am too young.
The job market is poor.
I am too old.
I have too many children.
My mate will not want me to.
I am afraid to get out of my present situation.
I owe too many bills.
I am too thin.
I do not have enough money.
I am not smart enough.
I am too fat.
I do not have a job.
Nobody likes me.
I live in a bad neighborhood.
I do not have a car.
What excuses have *you* used?

• Discuss the readings. Ask especially for other excuses they have used.

• This week we are going to talk about education, both formal and informal, or preparing to get a job, if that is what you want to do. Everyone has interests, skills, and talents. When you were a child, what did you tell people you wanted to be when you grew up? (Ask each one around the group.) . . . What kind of job would you most like to have *now*? . . . Can you get it with the education or training you already have? . . . What would you need to do first to try to get this job? . . . (learn more about it, then learn what you have to know to get it). Even if you cannot work right now, what can you do to feel better about yourself? . . . (work on your GED, sign up for a class at your local school). If you did not finish high school, what kinds of jobs can you get now? . . . (fast food, other minimum-wage jobs). What types of jobs do you have to take when you have little education? . . . (those that use your muscles more than your brain, such as digging ditches or other similar jobs). What does it take to get promoted to a better job? . . . (usually more education or some type of on-the-job training).

You need to set reasonable goals for yourself. You cannot start work as the president of the company, nor can you suddenly decide to become a brain surgeon "tomorrow." All jobs require step-by-step planning in order to turn your desire into a goal and your goal into reality. What would be *your* first step in getting the job you want? (Ask several group members.) . . . Your second step? . . . (Ask additional steps if desired.) Be sure what you want to do is something that is *possible* for you. If you are terrified of animals, you will not want to train to be a veterinarian. If you faint at the sight of blood, being a nurse is probably not a good choice. If you have three children and very little money, you will most likely not want to wait as long as it would take to become a doctor, unless your motivation is so strong you are willing to give up a lot in the present to get more in the future. (Time: 30 minutes.)

• This exercise is to help participants identify how they see themselves now and what they would like to change. You may not have time for this if the previous discussion lasts longer than the time allowed. (Time: 15 minutes.)

IF I WERE—

Have group members imagine what they would want to be if they were suddenly turned into an animal, a car, a flower, a bird, a food, or a building. Then have them describe *why* they made the choice that they did. For example, "If I were a building, I would be a cabin in the woods because I feel that lonely," or "If I were a flower I would be a rose, because roses are so beautiful." Go around the group for each topic. Then ask what they would *rather* be and why. This exercise is based on one in *100 Ways to Enhance Self-Concept in the Classroom*, by Jack Canfield and Harold Wells.

• Announce time for a break and food. Children may eat with adults if desired. (Time: 30 minutes.)

• Introduce the speaker. This speaker may be from a local junior college or university or a high school counselor. If no speaker is available and the facilitator must cover the topic, research should be done on nearby institutions or programs where group members can get their general equivalency diplomas (GEDs) or where they can get education beyond high school. Include costs; how, when, and where to enroll; how long they must attend; if financial assistance is available; and what types of courses are offered. A speaker should cover the same topics. (Time: 30 minutes.)

• An additional speaker from a local job-training organization or trade school can be used here. If the facilitator must continue, as much information should be gathered as possible on opportunities in the participants' area. State employment agencies and rehabilitation or retraining programs should be mentioned, and eligibilities explained. There are some government programs that offer temporary or permanent jobs, also. (Time: 20 minutes.)

• Depending on the time remaining, either read aloud, "What Things Can I Do Well?" or refer group members to their handbook to read how their interests can influence what job they might want.

WHAT THINGS CAN I DO WELL?

I like working with my hands and fixing things that break down. I like to build things and use tools. I like to take things apart or put them together. I will be happiest in a job that lets me touch things or make things with my hands or run a machine.

I am good at typing, keeping things in order, solving problems, and having set times to do things. I like to work with numbers and details. I will be happiest in a job that is organized, perhaps working with computers or numbers or in an office.

I am good at using things in new ways. I like to talk to people and find out things about them. I think in words or pictures and like to write things down. I will be happiest in a job that lets me do things my own way and express my feelings. I like to do things when I want to, not when I have to. I may want to be involved with music, drawing, painting, or writing. I may want to invent new things or find new ways to use old ones.

I enjoy talking to people and getting them to do things or buy things. I like to work with other people, not by myself. I like to help people or teach them. I will be happiest in a job selling things or working in a store or restaurant. I would be a good nurse, doctor, teacher, social worker, or person who helps others do something.

• Read aloud "Do You Want a Job?" Participants can follow in their handbooks.

DO YOU WANT A JOB?

When you *really* need a job for money to just *survive* from day to day you cannot be choosy. Many jobs are not exactly what you want, and they may not be ones you want to keep for the rest of your life but may be okay for a little while. Do your best there, but keep looking for something else. Remember, your goal is a job you can do, one you like, and one that makes you feel good about yourself.

Many jobs only require reading, writing, simple math, the ability to follow directions, talk to people, and learn new things from someone who shows you what to do.

You may also need to know how to drive a car. You can probably do most of those things now and find something to support yourself on your way to your *goal* job.

Choose your goal job; write down what it is and all of the steps you have to take to reach it. Do not choose something you know is impossible to reach, rather something you feel you can really do. How can you take those steps? You may need to get your GED, go to junior college, university, trade school, or get on-the-job training to learn new skills. Take one step at a time and have faith in your ability to reach your goal. It may take a while, but if you keep climbing the ladder, you will eventually reach the top. Then you will be prepared to get your goal job—the job you have always wanted!

• Distribute evaluation forms; have pencils available. Names are optional. Collect them facedown on one of the tables. (Time: 5 minutes.)

• Hold the Pretty Prize drawing. Be sure all group members are entered. The same person cannot win two weeks in succession. (Time: 5 minutes.)

• Do the Car Wash exercise if time allows.

Chapter 10

Week Eight: My Health

Goals for the Week Are:

1. To make participants aware of common health problems, risks, and ways to prevent illness.
2. To discuss serious illnesses and sexually transmitted diseases, including AIDS.
3. To explain the basic anatomy of both males and females and the reproductive process.

Materials Needed:

A Participant Handbook for each group member
Pens, felt-tip markers, and paper or notebook for sign-in
Name tags
Pencils for participants
Handouts on health issues, if you cannot arrange for a speaker
Chalkboard, flip chart, or large pad of drawing paper
Pretty Prize(s)

General good health, as well as preventive measures to avoid illness, is discussed this week. Depending on the ages and composition of the group, the facilitator should cover various topics. All ages need information on general good health habits as well as uncontrollable risk factors, such as age, gender, and race. Preventive measures such as immunizations and tests available to aid in early diagnosis of problems, as well as male and female anatomy, should be covered. Many group members may not have finished high school and never had instruction in basic biology. Some women who have borne children have little knowledge of the actual process of childbirth or what was happening inside their bodies while they were pregnant. Men may not understand either their own or women's bodies. Group members may not have enough medical knowledge to understand why they are given certain instructions by their doctor. The LAMS group should be a safe environment where they can ask the questions they have been afraid to ask their doctors for fear they would show their ignorance.

Health information should be tailored to the audience. If drugs and alcohol are important factors, much of the session should focus on those issues. Sexual behaviors, birth control, and sexually trans-mitted diseases should be discussed with many age groups. Con-doms can be obtained from your local health department and dis-tributed, if desired, and their use explained.

Having a speaker for this session is important, both for accurate information and for the added impact a medical person brings to the presentation. Speakers can be nurses, doctors, or other medical per-sonnel. School nurses could speak; public health departments might provide a speaker. Organizations such as the American Red Cross and various disease-related groups are also possibilities. Handouts are helpful, as the information is more likely to be remembered if something can be taken home and looked at later. There are many good videos available on medical subjects that could add to the speaker's presentation.

You should still begin the session with the usual group Affirma-tion for Week Eight, reading aloud, in unison.

Some general health questions can serve as a lead-in for the speaker. They are listed in the material for this week. This session will need to be tailored to your particular group, depending on the problems needing to be addressed and the ages of the group mem-bers. If necessary, the facilitator can conduct the session with help from videos or handouts, but it is more effective if a medical profes-sional presents the information.

Close the session as usual with evaluations, the Pretty Prize draw-ing, and the Car Wash exercise. Do not forget to include a graduation ceremony, despite the speaker, if this is someone's last week.

WEEK EIGHT: MY HEALTH

• After registration, give all new members a Participant Handbook and Pre-Lams Questionnaire to be completed and handed in at the end of the session.

• Introduce the facilitator(s), give a brief description of the LAMS program, and discuss housekeeping issues. (Time: 5 minutes.)

• Read the Affirmation aloud, in unison; participants should read from their handbooks. (Time: 5 minutes.)

> I choose to do everything I can to stay healthy.
> I deserve to take care of my own health as well as that
>   of my family.
> I will learn all I can about my body and how
>   to protect myself from illness.
> I will seek medical care when I need it and not wait
>   for things to "go away."
> I will learn to relax and take things easier, without
>   getting stressed over little things.

• You should have a speaker today—a nurse, doctor, or someone else with medical knowledge. Before the speaker begins, discuss the following questions (Time: 20 minutes):

> Today we are going to talk about your health, things you can do to help you stay well, and how your body works. How many of you neglect your own illnesses as unimportant, yet do something right away if someone else in the family gets sick?. . . How much do you know about health risks and what you can do to stay healthy? . . . Can any of you name a sexually transmitted disease? . . . (AIDS, syphilis, gonorrhea, chlamydia, genital warts). Do you do monthly breast self-examination? (And, yes, men can also get breast cancer.) . . . Men, do you do a regular examination of your testicles for unusual lumps? . . . Women, do you have yearly pap smears for possible cancer of the cervix or uterus? . . . If you are over forty,

do you have regular mammograms? . . . You should have a baseline mammogram done about age forty and yearly ones done after age 50. Can you tell me some of the dangers of smoking while pregnant? . . . What about drinking during pregnancy? . . . Do you have your blood pressure taken at least yearly and more often if you are overweight or in a high-risk group? . . . All of those things are important, and our speaker today, _____, can tell us much more about these and other medical subjects and answer any questions you may have.

• The speaker should address stress reduction; risk factors associated with age, sex, race, health habits, and genetics in certain conditions or diseases; family planning; prenatal care and childbirth; and immunizations. The facilitator should tell the speaker in advance what topics to address and if there are special topics, such as safer sex, risks of indiscriminate sex, condoms, or birth control. Drug or alcohol abuse may also need to be covered. (Time: 30 minutes.)

• Announce time for a break and food. Children may eat with adults if desired. (Time: 30 minutes.)

• The speaker should continue after break. A video could be shown as part of the presentation. *Things My Mother Never Told Me* is a very good video. A stress-reduction or relaxation exercise could also be used here. (Time: 45 minutes.)

• Distribute evaluation forms; have pencils available. Names are optional. Collect them facedown on one of the tables. (Time: 5 minutes.)

• Hold the Pretty Prize drawing. Be sure all group members are entered. The same person cannot win two weeks in succession. (Time: 5 minutes.)

• Do the Car Wash exercise. There may not be time if the speaker answers several questions. (Time: 5 minutes.)

Chapter 11

Week Nine: My Family

Goals for the Week Are:

1. To discuss "Poison" statements, IALAC, and do the "Spears and Cheers" exercise
2. To learn how things that happened to you as a child affect you today
3. To talk about spousal abuse

Materials Needed:

A Participant Handbook for each group member
Pens, felt-tip markers, and paper or notebook for sign-in
Name tags
Pencils for participants
Colored clay dough, shaped into a ball, for Spears and Cheers exercise
Toothpicks, plastic picks, or any small sticks, for Spears and Cheers
9-by-12-inch colored construction paper, one sheet for each group member, with IALAC written in large letters in the middle
Black wide-tip marker for printing the IALAC sheets
Chalkboard, flip chart, or large pad of drawing paper
Pretty Prize(s)

One of the main goals of the LAMS program is to help participants understand how childhood happenings influence their adult lives. "Poison" statements heard as children often cannot be totally forgotten. "You are *so* stupid" or "You are just like your mother" may have been heard from parents. "Why are you always late?" or "You can never get your work done on time" may have been heard from teachers. Group members heard those things so often they felt they were true, and many of them feel they are still true today.

Begin the group with the unison reading of the Affirmation for the week, with participants reading from their handbooks. There are no extra readings today, but there is a general discussion of "Poison" statements (demeaning remarks made by parents, teachers, or others from childhood). Mention IALAC, and ask if anyone knows what it means; then, tell them the letters stand for "I Am Lovable and Capable." Ask if they know what "Spears and Cheers" are (negative and positive statements from others).

The "Spears and Cheers" exercise illustrates with clay dough and toothpicks how hurtful remarks leave holes in self-esteem. Make a ball out of one can of clay dough (that represents self-esteem). Use either regular toothpicks, small sticks such as cut wooden matches, or plastic picks to make holes. Visible holes are important, so fairly large picks are best. The ball of clay dough is passed around the circle, as described in this week's material, and group members insert picks in the clay as they repeat "poison" statements they heard as children, such as "You are stupid," "You can't do anything right," or "You'll never amount to anything." Then the same picks are taken out, as per instructions, and participants are left with lots of "holes" in their "self-esteem" ball of clay. This is a very effective demonstration of what happens when children hear nothing but bad comments. The facilitator should caution the participants against making those kinds of remarks to their own children, lest they grow up feeling they are not worthwhile people.

This exercise has been used with child welfare board members, including businessmen and judges, and they found it as interesting and effective as LAMS participants do. These professionals had heard as many negative things as group members but were better able to overcome the holes in their self-esteem.

After discussion of the "Spears and Cheers" exercise, introduce the IALAC (I Am Lovable and Capable) activity. This demonstrates how self-esteem can be nibbled away by everyday happenings. Use the reading included in the material or make up another scenario more applicable to the makeup of the LAMS group being conducted. Prior to session meeting time, prepare sheets of colored construction paper with the letters IALAC written on them. Make enough for all group members and the facilitators. These sheets of paper represent self-esteem. When they are passed out to everyone, begin the reading, tearing pieces off the piece of paper when "Poison" statements are made. What is left at the end of the reading is what is left of positive self-image after a day of constant assaults and no positive reinforcement, either from within or without.

Other childhood issues are brought up, including past child abuse or having parents who were substance abusers. Changing yourself, instead of giving in to what others want you to be, is discussed. How to handle stress is another topic, as well as the tendency to blame others for things instead of taking responsibility for your own life.

Role-plays are set up to illustrate how "put-downs" can destroy self-esteem. Ask for volunteers, but be prepared to demonstrate if group members are timid about acting in front of everyone.

Rights, especially the right not to be abused by anyone, are addressed, as well as a little bit about the cycle of violence and how abusers often abuse and later apologize to try to make up for their behavior with love and presents. If there is a shelter nearby for women who have been abused, the facilitator may want to have their literature and telephone number available.

Finish the session with evaluations, the Pretty Prize drawing, and the Car Wash exercise if there is time.

WEEK NINE: MY FAMILY

• Register all new members and give each a Participant Handbook and Pre-LAMS Questionnaire to be completed and handed in at the end of the session.

• Introduce the facilitator(s), give a brief description of the LAMS program, and discuss housekeeping issues. (Time: 5 minutes.)

• Read the Affirmation aloud, in unison; participants should read from their handbooks. (Time: 5 minutes.)

> I choose to do everything I can to make my family
> a happy one.

I will remember IALAC, and I will not let others
destroy me with "poison" statements.
I will remember that what my parents or others told me
when I was small may not have been true.
I will think in "Cheers," not in "Spears."

• Hold up one of the IALAC sheets to be used later in the session. Ask if anyone knows what that means. Explain that it means "I Am Lovable and Capable." Do not explain it further at this time.

• Does anyone know what a "Poison" statement is? . . . It is something someone tells you that makes you feel terrible but is not necessarily true. Can you give me some examples? I will write them on the board as you call them out. . . . (You are stupid; you never do anything right; you will never learn; you will never amount to anything; I wish you had never been born.) Now we are going to do something that will help you understand how the things you heard as a child affect you even now. (Time: 10 minutes.)

• For the next exercise, make a ball of clay dough three to four inches in diameter (or contents of one regular-sized can). Hold up the ball to show the group. Explain as follows (Time: 15 minutes):

SPEARS AND CHEERS

I am going to pass this ball of clay dough around the group along with a box of toothpicks (or whatever you are using). When you get the ball, I want you to put a toothpick into it while repeating a "poison" statement you heard as a child—something that hurt you or was untrue. Then pass it on to the person next to you, so they can do the same. (Leader may begin, as an example, jabbing the ball with feeling while saying something, such as "You never do anything right.")

When the clay returns to the group leader, hold it up again with toothpicks intact. Do not explain beyond asking them what you have (a ball with toothpicks in it).

Now we will pass the ball to everyone in the group again. When you get it this time take *out* a toothpick, and say something you would have *liked* to have people say to you as a child. ("I love you" is often a choice; leader begins by taking out a toothpick and making a positive statement.)

When the ball is again returned, hold it up for everyone to see. Then discuss the following:

What do we have now? . . .What you are looking at is what happens to how you feel about yourself—your self-esteem—when you hear hurtful things. All of those remarks leave "holes," even when you are grown. What you need to do now is work on filling those "holes" with good comments. Remember those holes when you are speaking to your own children. Even if words are said in anger and without thought, they can leave wounds as surely as if they were shot from a bow and arrow. The old saying, "Sticks and stones may break my bones, but words can never hurt me" is far from true. Words *can* hurt, and the hurt can last for years. Which statements made you feel better, the "Spears" or the "Cheers?" . . . Can you remember some things that were said to you over and over that made you believe something about yourself today? . . . Have you thought about whether they were really true? . . .

• Next, introduce the IALAC exercise, which is another illustration of how self-esteem can be destroyed even in day-to-day happenings. This is based on an idea by Dr. William Glasser, which appeared in *100 Ways to Enhance Self-Concept in the Classroom*, by Canfield and Wells. They granted permission for the idea of IALAC to be shared, and the story to be changed as needed. (Time: 10 minutes.)

IALAC

Now we are going to do something else that shows how your self-esteem, or how you feel about yourself, can be destroyed. I am going to give all of you a sheet of colored paper with IALAC printed on it. Does anyone remember what that means? . . . (I Am Lovable and Capable.) Each one of us has our own internal "sign" (hold up your sign). The size of your sign changes during the day as people say things that make you feel bad or hurt your feelings. They may tease you, or reject you, or put you down, and each time they do a little piece of your "sign" is torn off. (Illustrate this by tearing off a corner of your sign.) Now I am going to read you a story about one mother's day, and I want you to tear off a piece of your sign every time you think she is going to have a tear in how she feels about herself. (Be as dramatic and realistic as you can be without overacting. You can change this story any way you want to or make up an entirely new story to fit your situation.)

> Joan is still lying in bed five minutes after the alarm goes off. Her husband comes in from the bathroom and says, "Are you *ever* going to get up? Do you have to be lazy *every* morning?" (rip) She struggles awake and gets out of bed. She goes to the bathroom to wash up. Her husband yells, "Hurry up, I have to get ready for work, you do not have to go anywhere." (rip) She goes downstairs to fix breakfast; the dishes are still dirty from last night. Her husband is right behind her, saying, "This kitchen is a mess, you never do *anything* around here." (rip) He forgot that the baby cried all evening, and he never offered to help. She starts making lunches. Her son says, "Mom, why do you never fix anything I like?" (rip) The kids leave for school. The phone rings; it is her mother. During the conversation she asks, "Why did you buy that new TV set? You know you could not afford to spend that money, but you never did learn to save anything." (rip) A little later her sister comes over to visit. She starts her usual "fat" speech by saying, "You must be gaining weight again, those pants are too tight across your backside." (rip) Now she walks into the kitchen and says, "Your dishes are *still* dirty? It is almost 10 o'clock." (rip) Joan answers the phone again. It is the department store. "Did you forget your bill again? This is the *second*

time we have had to call you." (rip) Her sister leaves, and she picks up the house a little, but it is getting late and she has to pack up the baby and go to the grocery store. Her cart accidentally hits a display, and everything falls to the floor; she tries to apologize, but the manager glares at her anyway. (rip) She gets to the checkout counter, balancing the baby on her hip. She is short $1.00 of what she needs to pay the bill. The lady behind her in line makes insulting remarks out loud. (rip) Soon after she arrives back home, her children return from school. Her teenaged daughter looks at her critically and says, "Mom, do you always have to wear such dumpy-looking clothes?" (rip) She did not look quite so dumpy before juggling the baby at the store. An hour later her husband comes in from work and says, "This house is a mess. What have you been doing all day—watching the soaps?" (rip) After supper she is watching her favorite TV show, but her husband and kids want to see something else, so they change the channel right in the middle of the show without asking if she was watching what was on. (rip) Then her husband asks if he has a clean shirt for tomorrow. She forgot she needed to wash one. He says, "You never remember anything important." (rip)

Hold up your sign and say, "Not much left, is there!" (Have the participants hold up their signs, so everyone can see what happened to Joan's self-esteem during the day.)

• It takes courage to be yourself; it takes courage to change. Not changing is easier, and it is easier to give in and do what other people want even when you really want to say "no." It is easier to give in to what your children want even when those wants are unreasonable. It is easier to forget you are a person, too, with rights of your own. You think you have to be "nice" so people will like you instead of reject or even *leave* you. You may be financially dependent on a man and afraid to be on your own, even though you may be living in an unhealthy or unhappy situation. You do not want him, your family, or your children to be "mad" at you, so you give up your right to be happy.

Do you have to have peace at any price? . . . Why? . . . What happened when you were a child that might make you feel that way? . . . What happens now? . . . What feelings do you have when you never get your own needs met? . . . (tiredness from "stuffing" feelings, depression, and anger). What things can you do to feel better?" . . . (exercise, walk, read, listen to music, do something nice for yourself). (Time: 15 minutes.)

• Announce time for a break and food. Children may eat with adults if desired. (Time: 30 minutes.)

• Do not blame others for everything. Quit resisting change. Do not use excuses that keep you in the same old rut, saying things such as, "I forgot; I overslept; I was too tired. Why do I need to change? Everything is okay this way. I cannot do that. It does not matter anyway; nobody reminded me." *You* are responsible for your own life, and you *can* make things better.

What are some of the things that happened to you when you were a child that affect the way you are today? Were you abused or neglected as a child? . . . If so, you did not have a very good example of how you should act today. If your parents hit you every time you did something even slightly wrong, even if you did not understand *why* it was wrong, then it is no wonder you did not learn other ways to discipline your own children. If your mother did not care if the house was dirty, you probably never learned how to keep a clean house. If she did not care where you were or what you did when you were a child, you may find it hard to properly watch your own children. If you were sexually abused, you were made to feel as if *you* were bad when really you were the *victim*, and the person who *abused* you was bad.

All of these past experiences may make you feel depressed, as if you are crying on the inside, or they may make you confused about what is happening in your family now. They may make you feel that you are a bad person or a bad parent. Just because these bad experiences were a part of your past, or even if they are happening now, it does not mean that your future is hopeless; you can learn new ways to behave, and it can be the beginning of something better for all of you.

We all cope with stress in different ways. Some people cry, some get angry and hard to be around, and some get physically ill. Others may turn to alcohol or drugs. Some just "give up" and do not even *try* to get past their problems. If you are ill, drunk, or high, people do not expect you to cope with things; others will have to take care of you and make decisions for you, or if things just drift on, the decisions will be made for you just because you take no action at all. Take some action. Hit a pillow, yell, or walk fast around the block, but do not hit some*body*. Accept what is happening if that is your only choice, or change things if you can, but do not just *sit there* and do nothing! (Time: 20 minutes.)

• Go around the group and ask again for some examples of "Poison" statements—things the group members heard while they were children—or read some off the board, if they were put there. (You are so stupid; you can never do anything right; you are so clumsy; you always act just like your father; you should be ashamed of yourself.) Do you remember what happens if you hear those kinds of comments all of the time when you are a child? . . . What if your husband or wife, or boyfriend or girlfriend says more of the same? . . . (Time: 10 minutes.)

ROLE-PLAYS

Ask for two volunteers to be a mother and child. Set up any situation where the child is being "put down by the mother" (for spilling something, getting bad grades, not cleaning their room properly).

Ask two more volunteers to be husband or boyfriend and wife or girlfriend in another "put-down" situation (wife did not clean the house to husband's satisfaction; husband left the bathroom a mess after shaving; wife did not have supper ready on time). (Time: 10 minutes.)

• The following exercise applies only to women and would need to be changed in some groups.

Now we need to talk about your rights as women. Call out some rights that you think you have, and I will write them on the board. . . . Here are some more. You have the *right* to be treated with respect. You have the *right* to express your opinions; you have the *right* to have feelings. You have the *right* to be listened to and taken seriously; you have the *right* to say "no" without feeling guilty, and you have the *right* to ask for what you want and need.

Nobody has the *right* to hit you, no matter what you do or say. You cannot *make* somebody mad; they *let* themselves get mad. Your partner cannot say, "If you had not _____, I would not have hit you." It is *not* your fault, no matter how many times he tries to tell you it is. Sure, he may apologize, beg, or even cry, and promise never to do it again, but that *does not* make it okay. If he hits you once, he will probably do it again unless he gets help from professionals. You have two choices—stay or leave. Whichever, think about it first, make plans, and do not decide in haste *unless* either you or your children are in real danger. If you are, call a friend, your family, the police, or a women's shelter, but get out of the house *immediately!*

The facilitator should give out telephone numbers for police, shelters in the area, or women's groups concerned with abuse. (Time: 10 minutes.)

• Distribute evaluation forms; have pencils available. Names are optional. Collect them facedown on one of the tables. (Time: 5 minutes.)

• Hold the Pretty Prize drawing. Be sure all group members are entered. The same person cannot win two weeks in succession. (Time: 5 minutes.)

• Do the Car Wash exercise if there is time.

Chapter 12

Week Ten:
My Financial Responsibility

Goals for the Week Are:

1. To learn basic budgeting using envelopes and play money
2. To learn how to shop for "specials"
3. To learn how to get the most for your shopping dollar
4. To play "Price Is Right" with generic and brand-name products

Materials Needed:

A Participant Handbook for each group member
Pens, felt-tip markers, and paper or notebook for sign-in
Name tags
Pencils for participants
A blank sheet of paper for each group member to write down income and expenses
Play money—you can buy money ranging from $1 to $20 bills in toy departments (often displayed with party favors), but you may need to cut some paper into bill-size sections and write larger denominations on them.
Either regular or business-size envelopes, several for each participant
Grocery store sale "flyers"
Canned or boxed food with "Nutrition Information" panels or an enlarged example
Grocery items, one brand-name and one generic for six products, for "Price is Right"

Cash register receipt for the grocery items, to check prices
Paper to keep track of bids on grocery items
Chalkboard, flip chart, or large pad of drawing paper

The topics for this week are budgeting and shopping. The budgeting taught in this session is very simple, not at all like what is found in budget books bought in stores. Grocery shopping is more complicated than it appears, and many group members have no idea of how to save money, buy nutritious food, or compare prices. By the end of this session, they should have learned the basics of budgeting and become more educated shoppers.

Begin the group by asking everyone to turn to the Affirmation in their handbooks, and then read it aloud, in unison. Do the exercise on acquiring unexpected money and what would be done with that money if it could be kept or had to be given away.

Depending on the makeup of your LAMS group, some participants may have barely enough money to cover the essentials of living, or they may only need to be more organized to be sure all their bills are paid. The envelope method is extremely simple, yet effective. Group members list all of their income and all of their bills on a sheet of paper. They receive, in play money, an amount equal to their monthly income, and then they place the amount of each bill in the labeled envelope. They can then see whether they have any money left and if so, try to discover what happens to the excess they should have at the end of the month. If they have more bills than income, they realize they may need to cut their spending. If they receive food stamp allotments, that money can also be divided equally for the four weeks they need to cover in order to avoid having more month than money, as often happens. What to do and where to go if you cannot pay a bill is discussed, as well as which bills are most important and should never be skipped. The play money needs to be returned to the leaders after the exercise (unless there is a large budget for your LAMS group!), but group members can keep the envelopes.

How to shop well and get the most for your money is also an important topic this week. A good smart-shopping exercise can be conducted by using weekly grocery flyers found in the newspaper or at local stores. Collect them for several weeks so you will have current ones as well as ones from holiday periods and different seasons of the year. Pass out several flyers to each group member. The leader should call out various products and have participants look in their flyers to find that product and compare prices at different stores. Mention products that are cheaper at certain seasons, such as turkeys at Thanksgiving and picnic supplies near the Fourth of July.

Much of the information on shopping is included in the handbooks so group members will be able to refer to it after the session is over. They can follow along as the leader shows how to read labels for nutritional value and how to read shelf prices in order to make price comparisons between products. Participants are given tips on buying other items besides groceries at the best possible prices and where and how to shop.

The session concludes with a "Price Is Right" game of comparing brand-name and generic products. Twelve products, six brand-name and six generic, are purchased in advance by the facilitator, then are bid on by group members, as is done in the "Price Is Right" game on TV. The closest bidder, without going over the price, gets to keep the product. Many group members are amazed to learn how much they can save on generic products; sometimes brand-name products cost twice as much. Some generic products are poorer quality, but many are indistinguishable from the more expensive items. There is no Pretty Prize today, as players in the "Price Is Right" get to keep the products they correctly bid on.

Do the evaluations and the Car Wash exercise if time permits. Always remember to work in graduation ceremonies whenever needed, as completion of the LAMS program is an important accomplishment for the participants.

WEEK TEN: MY FINANCIAL RESPONSIBILITY

• Register all new members and give each a Participant Handbook and Pre-LAMS Questionnaire to be completed and handed in at the end of the session.

• Introduce the facilitator(s), give a brief description of the LAMS program, and discuss housekeeping issues. (Time: 5 minutes.)

• Read the Affirmation aloud, in unison; participants should read from their handbooks. (Time: 5 minutes.)

> I will learn to budget my money so it will cover my
>   expenses for the month.
> I choose to pay all my bills and to be sure they are paid
>   on time.
> I choose to be a careful shopper and get the most I can
>   for my money.
> I will prepare sensible meals and not eat only "junk food."
> I will learn to have a positive attitude even when things
>   are difficult for me.

• The following is a thought-provoking exercise with questions for the group. Based on an idea originally presented in *100 Ways to Enhance Self-Concept in the Classroom*, by Canfield and Wells. (Time: 15 minutes.)

INHERITANCE

> Since today we are talking about money, I want all of you to imagine you have been left $10,000 by a long-lost relative—money you were not expecting. How would you spend it? . . . (individually ask everyone in the group).
> Now a more difficult question. What if you were given the money but were required to give it away immediately to someone outside your family, under terms of the will. Who would you give it to and why? . . . (again ask everyone).

BUDGETING EXERCISE

Pass out sheets of paper and pencils to participants. Have them list their total monthly income at the top and below that their bills and the approximate amount paid each month. Have them count any regular expenses such as diapers, gasoline, or cigarettes as bills, also. Then distribute play money (this is sold as party favors and looks like real money, only smaller and printed on one side) in the amount of their income. Plain paper, cut to size, should be used to make larger denominations, as $20 bills are the largest sold. It saves time if the money is divided into $50 and $100 stacks beforehand. Give each participant one plain envelope for each bill they have listed.

Next, instruct group members to label each envelope with the amount of one bill. They are to put that amount of play money into the envelope; they should continue to do that with all of their bills (change can be made by the facilitator). Some may come out with extra money and some with not enough to cover their bills. Some will be surprised at the amount left over, and it will be a puzzle to try to find out where the extra money goes each month. Part of this is most likely the amount spent on soft drinks, chips, and other nonessentials during the month. Participants may want to expand this exercise and project amounts needed for clothing and other budget items.

Those who receive food stamps or allowances and have problems with running out before the end of the month may wish to divide the total into weekly amounts, also. Explain that larger amounts might need to be spent at the first part of the month for staples, then lesser amounts for perishable groceries bought later in the month.

After group members have completed the exercise, and everyone has a list of bills in front of them, discuss the following:

> Which are your most important bills? . . . (rent, utilities except telephone, food, diapers, or formula). Which can be put off if necessary? . . . (telephone, nonessential items). What can you do if you cannot pay your rent? . . . (list area resources that give emergency rental assistance). What if you cannot pay a utility bill? . . . (contact the utility company, or an emergency resource). Where can you get emergency food, formula, or diapers? . . . (list area resources). What kinds of activities can you do for fun if there is little or no money left after you pay the bills? . . . (go to the park, window-shop at the mall, ride bikes if available, go to a dollar movie, rent a video and make popcorn, watch TV).

This is very basic budgeting, but it has been extremely helpful to participants. Some had no idea how to budget money to cover expenses for the entire month. They can take the labeled envelopes home, but the play money should be collected for reuse. (Time: 35 minutes.)

• Announce time for a break and food. Children may eat with adults if desired. (Time: 30 minutes.)

SMART-SHOPPING EXERCISE

Collect weekly flyers listing the specials at local grocery stores. Have enough so each group member can have at least two. Most should be fairly current, but keep some from holidays and special seasons.

Pass out two or three flyers to each participant. Call out a product, such as ground beef or potatoes, and let group members search their flyers for any listing. If they find the product, they are to call out its price. Compare various store prices, and discuss why that product may be on sale for less. Continue searching for several different products.

Describe *loss leaders*—products put on sale for possibly less than cost to bring in business. These appear on the front of the flyer to attract attention. They also may be a special promotion by the manufacturer to introduce a new product or stimulate sales. If shoppers went to every store and bought *just* those products, they could save quite a bit, but the stores are counting on them buying other things so they can make a profit. Some stores have certain limits or added dollar amounts that must be bought in order to get the sale price. Stores that have triple coupons or other special "come-ons" have to make up the money they spend by charging higher prices. The grocery business has a very small profit margin, sometimes as low as one percent, so every penny counts. Participants should compare stores and find one that best fits their needs and pocketbook.

Discuss *where to shop.* Avoid small stores in poorer neighborhoods; they have the highest prices. If at all possible, go to a large chain grocery store or warehouse-type store in a suburban area. These will have lower prices. Why do stores in poorer neighborhoods often have higher prices? . . . (They know customers have limited transportation to leave the area so will have to pay whatever is charged; they have higher theft and vandalism rates, so upkeep is more expensive.)

Discuss *how to shop*. Check sizes and prices per ounce. Grocery stores now have shelf labels that list unit or ounce prices (bring or make a sample shelf label). The large economy or family sizes are not always the cheapest; sometimes two smaller sizes, especially if they are on sale, may be cheaper. Often store brands of identical products may cost less than half the amount of brand-name ones. Store brands and generics are the same quality in most cases and are packed by the same processors as brand-name foods. Occasionally the lower-priced foods are not as uniform in size or as tasty, but at least try them; many are equal in taste and appearance. Some generic products, such as salad oil, mustard, or black pepper, are indistinguishable from brand-name products.

Explain how *cooking from scratch saves money*. Every step the processor does before a product is sold makes it cost more. Sometimes the time saved is worth the extra cost, but buying ready-to-serve food means less money that can be spent on something else.

Give examples of budget *stretchers*. Rice, beans, macaroni, spaghetti, and noodles, mixed with meats, sauces, and seasonings are much cheaper than ready-prepared "helpers," which must have meat added. Cake mixes have been around so long and are so convenient that prices are equal to, or even less, than "scratch" cakes.

Discuss *staples*. Ask if any group members know what "staples" are . . . (products you *must* have to be able to cook, such as sugar, salt, flour, and oil). These should always be on hand and be immediately replaced as they run out. Canned foods also keep well and can be kept for a longer time. Shopping should be done on a weekly basis if possible, certainly not day by day, as every trip to the store adds to the temptation to buy expensive or "junk" foods. Long-lasting, high-protein foods such as beans and peanut butter are good buys and are nutritious. Items such as bread, milk and other dairy products, eggs, and other perishables have to be purchased throughout the month. Making out weekly menus and using advertisements to see what is on sale, helps save money and makes shopping easier. Try to feed your family a healthy, balanced diet.

Explain *label reading*. Hold up a can of food with nutritional label visible and talk about what is listed on the label. (The first ingredient is the one contained in most quantity, continuing in descending order; also vitamins, fat, carbohydrates, etc.) Explain why this information is valuable to the consumer.

Discuss *coupons.* Ask if group members use coupons. . . . (they save money, almost all stores accept them, they are free to you). If not, why not? . . .

Discuss *seasonal specials.* Explain buying things "in season." Do not buy watermelon in January; buy it in the summertime when it is grown. Ask when turkeys would be cheapest. . . . (near Thanksgiving and Christmas). When would picnic foods be cheapest? . . . (Fourth of July or other summer holidays). When are fresh vegetables cheapest? . . . (summertime, when they are grown). When are local Farmer's Markets open? . . . (when local produce is being harvested). Mention that food stamps are accepted in some farmer's markets. Ask if anyone can think of other seasonal specials. . . .

Discuss *shopping for clothing and other items.* Ask where to get bargains on clothing or other items. . . . (Goodwill, Salvation Army stores, garage sales, flea markets, discount or outlet stores, end-of-season sales). Ask if group members trade outgrown clothing with others who may have younger or older children than their own. . . . This can save considerable money if the clothing is in usable condition. Watch for shoe sales, as shoes usually cannot be handed down. (Time: 30 minutes.)

"PRICE IS RIGHT" EXERCISE

This replaces the Pretty Prize this week, as several group members will win grocery products to take home.

Prepurchase about twelve grocery items, half generic or store brands and half identical, brand-name products. Select items with large price differences. Some possibilities are mustard, black pepper, salad oil, soaps, and canned tomatoes. Do not select items where there are obvious preferences (breakfast cereals, salad dressings) or quality differences (paper towels, toilet tissue). Another good comparison is the amount of juice in drink boxes versus cans of the same drink. Beans or rice are good examples of low-cost nutritious foods. Have the cash register slip available to check prices. This is an exercise where an assistant is very helpful.

Draw three names from the "Pretty Prize" bag and choose the first product. (As an alternative method of play, teams could be selected to bid.) Hold the product up and describe it, including weight or ounces contained. Let each of the three participants bid on the product and record their bids. The one closest, but under the price, is the winner. If all overbid, they must bid again. The winner gets to keep that product. Then choose three more names. They bid on the companion product, noting whether it is brand-name or generic, since the brand-name products will cost more.

Draw three more names and continue until all of the products have been given out, putting names already drawn back in the bag after each round.

This is a real learning experience, as many participants have never noted the tremendous price differences in the same products; some prices are double for the same amount of product or less. (Time: 25 minutes.)

• Distribute evaluation forms; have pencils available. Names are optional. Collect them facedown on one of the tables. (Time: 5 minutes.)

• Do the Car Wash exercise if there is time.

Chapter 13

Week Eleven:
My Homemaking Skills

Goals for the Week Are:

1. To learn participants most- and least-liked foods
2. To present information on nutrition and meal preparation, either by a speaker or the facilitator
3. To request that favorite recipes be brought for inclusion in a cookbook

Materials Needed:

A Participant Handbook for each group member
Pens, felt-tip markers, and notebook or paper for sign-in
Name tags
Pencils for participants
A blank sheet of paper for each group member to record food likes and dislikes
Chalkboard, flip chart, or large pad of drawing paper
Pretty Prize(s)

If at all possible, obtain a speaker on nutrition. The local Department of Agriculture should have an Extension Service that might provide a speaker, or possibly a home economics teacher in a local high school or college could speak. If the facilitator must present the information, he or she can obtain it in libraries and through the

Department of Agriculture. Many food manufacturers also have printed nutritional information that can be obtained at little or no cost. Information needs to be presented on low-cost meal preparation, nutrients necessary for a healthy diet, and what quantities of different foods are required daily. If desired, information on home decorating could also be included this week or during one of the other two homemaking sessions. Tailor the session to the particular interests of your group.

Have all group members turn in their handbooks to the Affirmation for the week. Read it aloud, in unison. Next, the facilitator should read "Finish Every Day," while participants follow along in their books.

For the "Likes and Dislikes" exercise every group member needs paper and pencil. Have them list their favorite foods on the left side and their least-liked foods on the right. Pass the papers back and forth until they are thoroughly scrambled, then read each aloud, as everyone tries to guess the person who wrote that list. This leads into the topic for today—nutrition.

Introduce the speaker, if there is one, giving some information about his or her qualifications. If a speaker cannot be located, the facilitator can present the program.

Ask group members at break time if they have recipes that are family favorites. Ask them to bring them next week so a cookbook can be compiled on the third Homemaking Skills week. The facilitator will have to augment the recipes at first, but after presenting Week Eleven several times, there will be an increasing collection from participants in the group.

Continue with the speaker after break. If you have kitchen facilities, the speaker may wish to prepare a full meal, demonstrating healthy foods that are economical to fix. If a meal is prepared, the break may need to come at the end of the session, but do give a bathroom break halfway through the time period.

Finish the session with evaluations, the Pretty Prize drawing (possibly including something such as measuring spoons or cups in addition to beauty products), and the Car Wash exercise if there is still time.

WEEK ELEVEN: MY HOMEMAKING SKILLS

• After registration, all new members get a Participant Handbook and Pre-LAMS Questionnaire to be completed and handed in at the end of the session.

• Introduce the facilitator(s), give a brief description of the LAMS program, and discuss housekeeping issues. (Time: 5 minutes.)

• Read the Affirmation aloud, in unison; participants should read from their handbooks. (Time: 5 minutes.)

> I am a creative and worthwhile person even though
>   I make mistakes.
> I will take care of my family's health and well-being
>   and make my home a happy, comfortable place.
> I will learn to say "I can" even when my fear
>   wants me to say "I cannot."
> I will remember that I have the power to change my life.

• The facilitator should read aloud "Finish Every Day," which is paraphrased from a poem by Ralph Waldo Emerson. Group members should follow along in their handbooks.

FINISH EVERY DAY

> Finish every day and be done with it.
> You have done what you could.
> Some mistakes may have been made;
> Forget them as soon as you can.
> Tomorrow is a new day.
> Begin it with peace and happiness and feeling
>   too well to worry about yesterday.
> This day is good, with its own hopes and joys,
>   and it is too rich a gift to waste a moment on yesterdays.

• Do the "Likes and Dislikes" exercise. Give each group member a sheet of paper and a pencil. Instruct participants to fold their papers in half vertically. On the left side, ask them to write "Likes" at the top. On the right side, "Dislikes." Have each person list the five foods they like most and least. Then exchange papers until they are thoroughly scrambled. Have each person take turns reading aloud all the "Likes" and "Dislikes" on their paper. Participants then guess who wrote each list. This is a good get-acquainted game, and it also introduces the topic of this session—food and nutrition. (Time: 15 minutes.)

• Introduce the speaker. Arrange for a speaker if at all possible. The Department of Agriculture has an Expanded Nutrition Program through their local extension service in most areas. They have a several-hour series which can be presented over three weeks, with a graduation certificate awarded at the end. This covers proper nutrition, low-cost meal preparation, basic foods, vitamins and minerals, and healthy eating. If the facilitator does not have access to such a program, a speaker could be obtained through a local school's home economics department, or by contacting a local hospital dietician. The facilitator could also do research in a local library. Some food manufacturers have nutritional material available at little or no cost, and the Department of Agriculture has many pamphlets and bulletins that can be ordered. Handouts on the food pyramid of basic nutritional needs should be obtained if at all possible. If you are unable to fill three weeks on homemaking subjects, the LAMS program can be shortened to twelve weeks by having only one week on nutrition and combining the "My Goals" and "Celebration" weeks. Be sure to include at least one week on homemaking and food, as it is an important part of the LAMS curriculum.

Each week, with the Expanded Nutrition Program, the home economist-demonstrator cooks a one-dish meal for the group while talking about purchase and preparation of food and healthy eating habits (a full-course meal could be prepared if facilities are available). The emphasis is on saving money while feeding the family well. Questions are answered about how to get children to eat foods that are good for them, the amounts needed for good health, and the basic food groups. The facilitator could follow the same pattern if he or she is presenting the material. (Time: 35 minutes.)

• Announce time for a break. Drinks are available, but food today is served at the end of the session due to the speaker and required preparation time. (Time: 15 minutes.)

• Ask group members if they have favorite recipes they prepare at home, something simple and well-liked by their family. Most have some to share. Ask them to bring them next week so a cookbook can be put together on the third week of the homemaking series with their recipes included. (A good collection will eventually be acquired through contributions from each group, together with recipe handouts and some old favorites from recipe books.) (Time: 5 minutes.)

• Have the speaker continue with his or her presentation. (Time: 35 minutes.)

• Take a break to serve and eat the food that was prepared. (Time: 25 minutes.)

• Distribute evaluation forms; have pencils available. Names are optional. Collect them facedown on one of the tables. (Time: 5 minutes.)

• Hold the Pretty Prize drawing. Be sure all group members are entered. The same person cannot win two weeks in succession. (Time: 5 minutes.)

• Do the Car Wash exercise if there is time.

Chapter 14

Week Twelve: Second Week, Homemaking

Goals for the Week Are:

1. To imagine the "perfect" meal
2. To present additional topics on food and nutrition
3. To include a home-decorating or craft project

Materials Needed:

A Participant Handbook for each group member
Pens, felt-tip markers, and notebook or paper for sign-in
Name tags
Pencils for participants
A copy of the "Spice List" for each group member (in their handbooks)
Ten small glass or plastic jars filled with small amounts of various spices and herbs for the "Smell-A-Spice" game (See instructions for the exercise.)
Craft or special supplies needed for any additional project for this session
Chalkboard, flip chart, or large pad of drawing paper
Pretty Prize(s)

This is the second week concerning homemaking skills. Continue with a speaker if the three-week series is planned. A craft or home-decorating project could be included this week if desired. If there is an upcoming holiday, the facilitator may want to use that for the theme.

Start with the Affirmation for Week Twelve; read aloud, in unison. Group members should read from their handbooks. The facilitator should then read aloud "Family Rules" as everyone follows along.

Ask if anyone brought recipes this week, and collect them. Again remind them to bring recipes next week for the cookbook.

The first exercise involves distributing paper and pencil to all the group members so they can write down their concept of the "perfect" meal. Cost is not important, but they need to decide where they would want to eat (desert island, Cancún, Paris) and who they would share their meal with. Ask each participant to tell the group what her meal would be.

The speaker should be introduced, either the same person as last week or a different person or topic. A meal should again be prepared but can be done by the facilitators if the topic is not food this week. If preparation of a meal is part of what is presented, the halftime break should be short, with the meal eaten at the end of the session.

After break, play the "Smell-A-Spice" game. Fill small jars with about a teaspoon of various spices and herbs. A possible list follows in the directions for the session. The handbook has a checklist for this game, and group members write the number of the jar next to the listed spice they think it contains. This is fun and teaches "salt and pepper" cooks to experiment with new tastes. At the end of the activity, give possible uses for each of the spices and what foods usually contain them. Prizes of cans or bottles of spices can be given to the participants who make the most right choices.

Continue with a speaker or a presentation of some other homemaking project. If your session is near a holiday, a craft project could be completed during this time.

Finish with evaluations, the Pretty Prize drawing (connected with the topic for this week), and the Car Wash exercise if time remains.

WEEK TWELVE: SECOND WEEK, HOMEMAKING

• After registration, all new members get a Participant Handbook and Pre-LAMS Questionnaire to be completed and handed in at the end of the session.

• Introduce the facilitator(s), give a brief description of the LAMS program, and discuss housekeeping issues. (Time: 5 minutes.)

• Read the Affirmation aloud, in unison; participants should read from their handbooks. (Time: 5 minutes.)

> I am okay as I am; I do not have to be perfect.
> I will learn to love myself, as I cannot learn to love others
>   unless I do.
> I will learn as much as I can so that I can help myself
>   and others.
> I am in control of my own life.

• The facilitator should read aloud "Family Rules." The original author is unknown. Participants should follow along in their handbooks.

FAMILY RULES

> If you sleep in it—make it up.
> If you wear it—hang it up.
> If you eat out of it—put it in the sink.
> If you step on it—wipe it off.
> If you open it—close it.
> If you empty it—fill it up.
> If it rings—answer it.
> If it howls—feed it.
> If it cries—love it.

• Ask if anyone brought favorite recipes today for next week's cookbook. Collect them to copy later. Remind participants again to bring their favorites next week.

• Do the "Perfect Meal" exercise. Ask participants to imagine they could have the "perfect" meal served to them. Cost is not important. Where would they be, what would they eat, and who would they share it with? Ask each participant individually for their choices. (Time: 15 minutes.)

• Introduce the speaker, who should continue with topics on nutrition. Another economical meal should be prepared. (Time: 40 minutes.)

• Announce time for a break. Drinks are available. Food will be served at the end of the session due to speaker and preparation time. (Time: 15 minutes.)

• Play the "Smell-A-Spice" game. Many women do not use spices or herbs in cooking, only basic salt and pepper. This will introduce them to a broader selection of flavorings. (Time: 15 minutes.)

Before group, fill ten small glass or plastic jars (baby food jars, for example) with small amounts of various spices and herbs. Some seasonings with distinctive odors are: cinnamon, nutmeg, cloves, chili powder, garlic salt or powder, onion salt or powder, oregano, paper saturated with vanilla, sage, celery seed, pepper, and dill. Others could replace the ones listed. Number the jars one through ten. Be sure to write down which jar contains which spice as you number them.

Prepare a list of all the spices and herbs used as samples, plus a few extras. Do not list them in numerical order. Leave a short space after each for participants to write the number of the sample they think matches, as follows:

SPICE LIST

Chili powder ___
Vanilla ___
Green pepper ___
Cinnamon ___
Black pepper ___
Allspice ___
Poultry seasoning ___
Celery seed ___
Oregano ___
Basil ___

Sage ___
Garlic salt or powder ___
Cloves ___
Dill ___
Onion salt or powder ___
Nutmeg ___

Have participants turn to the Spice List in their handbooks. Be sure everyone has a pencil. Pass the samples in numerical order to every person. As they smell each spice, they mark the number of their choice on the list. After everyone has finished, read the correct choices. Describe their possible uses in recipes. The person who correctly identified the most wins a prize—a bottle or can of a spice or herb. Have two or three prizes available in case of ties.

• Have the speaker continue, or the facilitator can include information on home decoration. Research magazines or books for simple, inexpensive decorating tips. Another choice might be a simple craft project (picture, decorated wreath, Easter basket) possibly associated with an upcoming holiday. (Time: 15 minutes.)

• Take time for a break to eat the prepared food. (Time: 30 minutes.)

• Distribute evaluation forms; have pencils available. Names are optional. Collect them facedown on one of the tables. (Time: 5 minutes.)

• Hold the Pretty Prize drawing. Be sure all group members are entered. The same person cannot win two weeks in succession. (Time: 5 minutes.)

• Do the Car Wash exercise if there is time.

Chapter 15

Week Thirteen:
Third Week, Homemaking

Goals for the Week Are:

1. To prepare cookbooks from recipes brought by participants
2. Continue with speaker on nutrition, food preparation, or other homemaking subjects

Materials Needed:

A Participant Handbook for each group member
Pens, felt-tip markers, and notebook or paper for sign-in
Name tags
Pencils for participants
Plain, colored, pocket folders or file folders
Women's magazines with pictures of food
Glue
Scissors
Recipes, on separate pages
Chalkboard, flip chart, or large pad of drawing paper
Pretty Prize(s)

This is the third week on homemaking. Continue with the Expanded Nutrition Program or invite another speaker. The session begins with the Affirmation, read aloud and in unison. Group members read from their handbooks.

The main activity this week will be making a cookbook. Group members will cut food pictures from old magazines and glue them individually or as a collage, to a file or pocket folder. They could also be collected, hole-punched, and kept in notebooks if desired.

Copy any recipes brought by group members; add handouts from the speaker or other sources and a few recipes from cookbooks or the facilitator's own family favorites. The collection will grow larger as more people go through the LAMS program. Emphasize recipes that are simple and economical to prepare. The facilitator should prepare one cookbook in advance, as an example to be followed.

Continue with a speaker on nutrition and food or any other related topic. Prepare a meal as usual, either made by the facilitator or the speaker if that is part of the program. This week can be planned by the leader or by the group. Each succeeding Week Thirteen could be the same, or the topic could vary depending on the makeup of the LAMS group and their particular interests. If the Expanded Nutrition Program is being presented by the Extension Service, the group members will finish a basic number of hours and get a certificate of completion. This can be awarded during this session, but if it requires preparation time, it can be done during the Celebration week.

Close the session with evaluations, the Pretty Prize drawing, and the Car Wash exercise if time remains.

WEEK THIRTEEN: THIRD WEEK, HOMEMAKING

• After registration, all new members get a Participant Handbook and Pre-LAMS Questionnaire to be completed and handed in at the end of the session.

• Introduce the facilitator(s), give a brief description of the LAMS program, and discuss housekeeping issues. (Time: 5 minutes.)

• Read the Affirmation aloud, in unison; participants should read from their handbooks. (Time: 5 minutes.)

> I am not perfect, as nobody is perfect.
> I will do my best and be the best person I can be.
> I will love myself as I am and not feel I always fall short
>   and need changing.
> I will learn all I can in order to take care of myself
>   and my family.

• Prepare the cookbooks. Provide file or pocket folders to participants. The materials needed are women's magazines with pictures of food, scissors, and glue. Have participants cut out pictures of foods from magazines and glue them to the front and back of plain, colored folders. Ask for recipe contributions from the group, as was done the past two weeks. Make copies of any new submissions. Provide each LAMS participant with copies of recipes collected from past groups, the present group, and other family favorites. Handouts from the past two weeks and this week should also be placed in the folder. These can be hole-punched and fastened or left loose in the pockets. The facilitator should have a completed book as an example. (Time: 25 minutes.)

• Introduce the speaker who will discuss food, nutrition, or some other homemaking topic. A meal should be prepared as part of the presentation. (Time: 25 minutes.)

• Take a short break. Drinks are available. Food will be served at the end of the session due to preparation time. (Time: 15 minutes.)

• Have the speaker continue. (Time: 45 minutes.)

• Announce time for a break to eat the prepared food. (Time: 20 minutes.)

• Distribute evaluation forms; have pencils available. Names are optional. Collect them facedown on one of the tables. (Time: 5 minutes.)

• Hold the Pretty Prize drawing. Be sure all group members are entered. The same person cannot win two weeks in succession. (Time: 5 minutes.)

• Do the Car Wash exercise if time allows.

Chapter 16

Week Fourteen: My Goals

Goals for the Week Are:

1. To identify goals through making a collage
2. To learn how to set reachable goals for your life
3. To learn how to achieve those goals

Materials Needed:

A Participant Handbook for each group member
Pens, felt-tip markers, and notebook or paper for sign-in
Name tags
Pencils for participants
Varied magazines for a collage of goals
Glue
Scissors
One sheet of 12-by-18-inch white or colored paper for each
  participant
Chalkboard, flip chart, or large pad of drawing paper
Pretty Prize(s)

During this session, group members are to make a collage of their goals. Some may never before have considered what they want to accomplish in their lifetime or thought that they were capable of reaching any goals.

Begin with the Affirmation, which addresses goal-setting. Group members should turn in their handbooks to the Affirmation for Week Fourteen, and read it aloud, in unison. The facilitator should then read "Changing" aloud, as participants follow along in their handbooks.

The game "Hand-Eye-What?" (to point to the proper body part) illustrates how goals we set can be easily sidetracked.

For the collage, the leader will need to give each group member some old magazines, scissors, and a sheet of 12-by-18-inch paper. Have a sample completed or use samples from past groups. They can use pictures, words, or both to illustrate goals they have for the future. They then explain their choices to the group.

After the break, discuss winners and losers, as explained in the material for this week. Have group members call out some positive affirmations to be written on the board.

"The River," a song by Garth Brooks, is used next. This is played on a cassette player after telling the group to listen to the message the song conveys. Any song or poem could be used here, as long as it illustrates the importance of setting goals. Mixing presentations to use all five senses is an important part of LAMS, as everyone learns differently. It also varies the sessions so those attending do not get bored.

Following an analysis of the song, participants learn how to set reachable goals and finally, the steps needed to achieve them. Ask each group member what steps are involved in reaching the goal he or she most wants to achieve. Goal-setting is one of the key steps in learning to take control of your own life and realizing that everyone has the potential to succeed.

The last activity is a relaxation exercise. One is included in today's material, or you may wish to compose your own or use one from another source. Many group members have never been conscious of how they actually *feel*, whether they are tense or relaxed. This can be a new experience and may put them in touch with themselves so they realize they are persons with feelings, desires, and goals—that they are unique and special.

The session is concluded with evaluations, the Pretty Prize drawing, and the Car Wash exercise.

WEEK FOURTEEN: MY GOALS

• After registration, all new members get a Participant Handbook and Pre-LAMS Questionnaire to be completed and handed in at the end of the session.

• Introduce the facilitator(s), give a brief description of the LAMS program, and discuss housekeeping issues. (Time: 5 minutes.)
• Read the Affirmation aloud, in unison; participants should read from their handbooks. (Time: 5 minutes.)

> I am all right as I am even though I am not perfect.
> Mistakes are things I wish I had done differently
>   or things I did not do that I wish I had done.
> I will learn from my mistakes so I will not make
>   the same ones over and over.
> I will forgive myself for the mistakes I have made
>   and go on with my life.
> I will set new goals and not be discouraged by past failures.
> I will believe in myself.

• Read "Changing" aloud. Participants should follow along in their handbooks.

CHANGING

> Think about your life the way it is today. If you want it to be different, you must believe that *you* are the one who can change it. Life does not just "happen" to you; you *make* it happen.

> Nobody can *stop* you from changing your life.
> Nobody can *make* you change your life.

> Only you know how you want to change it.
> You have to begin and change it step by step.

Discuss the reading if desired; it is the preview of the content for the week.

• Play the "Hand-Eye-What?" game, which is based on "This is My Nose" in *The New Games Book* (p. 27), edited by Andrew Fluegelman. Give the following explanation (Time: 10 minutes):

> Now we are going to play a game that is difficult because it goes against everything you learned as a child. When you were little, your parents wanted you to point to your eye or your mouth when they asked you where it was. Today, we are going to do that, but when you point to your body part, you are going to call it another part. For instance, you might say "this is my ear" while pointing to your eye. Your goal is to have the person following you name a different part than the one you point to, but she may not follow through. She may forget and go back to what she learned as a child. The person following you points to the part you named but names yet another part. She may say "this is my eye" while pointing to her elbow. Continue around the group this way, always pointing to the named part but calling it something else.

The facilitator may want to begin the game to demonstrate how it is played. It illustrates how goals sometimes get sidetracked even though intentions were good.

• Make a collage of goals. The materials needed are magazines, scissors, glue, and one sheet of 12-by-18-inch paper for each group member. Distribute several magazines, scissors, glue, and paper to each participant. Instruct them to cut pictures and words from the magazines that illustrate things they would like to have or do in the future and then glue them into a collage of their goals. Pictures and words can be overlapped or arranged in any way desired. The facilitator may want to have a completed collage (or several from past groups) as an example. When all have finished, ask each participant to explain his or her picture. (Time: 40 minutes.)

• Announce time for a break and food. Children can eat with adults if desired. (Time: 30 minutes.)

• Do you think you are a winner? Winners follow through on what they say they will do. Losers only make promises. Winners listen.

Losers just wait until it is their turn to talk. Winners do more than their job. Losers say, "I only work here." Winners respect those who know more than they do and try to learn from them. Losers try to show them up for what they do not know. In LAMS you are learning to be a winner. Saying good things to yourself, and learning to believe them, can make you a winner. We begin every LAMS session with a positive affirmation—something that makes you feel better about yourself. You should repeat such affirmations to yourself every day. Write them on a piece of paper and put them on the bathroom mirror or on the refrigerator door—anyplace where you will see them many times during the day. When you believe you are a good person and in control of your life, you can plan ahead and set goals. Your thinking changes from believing you can do nothing to realizing that you can do almost anything. What you tell yourself can change your life. I want you to call out some positive affirmations—good things to tell yourself—and I will write them on the board. . . . (I love myself; I can say "no" without guilt; I am proud of myself; I am smart; I have rights). Forget all of the bad comments you have been saying to yourself for years. Many of those are leftovers from your childhood. Think only in positives and expect yourself to be the very best person you can be. Remember—what you *think* you can do, you *can*, even though it may take hard work. Do you let others control your life? . . . What is your reward, or payoff, for allowing them to do this? . . . (they will like me, they will not get mad at me). How can you set goals for yourself if you allow others to make decisions for you? . . . (Time: 15 minutes.)

• Play the song "The River," by Garth Brooks from the cassette, *Ropin' the Wind*. Another song or poem could be used here or anything with a similar message of the importance of setting goals. (Time: 10 minutes.)

> I am going to play "The River," by Garth Brooks. I want you to listen closely to the words, so you can tell me what they mean. After the song is played, ask the following questions: What did you think the message of the song was? . . . (setting goals; keeping yourself pointed toward what you want to do; not letting anything stop you). Do you know how to set goals for yourself? . . .

• What is your first step in setting a goal? . . . (Decide what you really want.) *Believe* that you can reach that goal. (Do not decide to do something you know nothing about; you will have a hard time imagining yourself doing it.) Be sure you do not have limitations that will keep you from reaching your goal. If you faint at the sight of blood, becoming a nurse is probably not a good choice. If you have a back problem, you cannot be a weight lifter. Be sure it is a goal you can reach by yourself without the help of others, unless they are willing to help. Maybe your husband will care for your children while you attend school. You need to reach your goal one step at a time. Do not plan to be a brain surgeon "tomorrow." Write down what you want to do and all of the things it will take to get there. For instance, if you want to be a teacher, you will need to find out what education you need; get your high school equivalency diploma (GED) if necessary; locate a college that has a program for teaching; find out how many classes you will need and how long you will have to go to school; apply for a loan or grant if necessary; register; finish the first, second, third, and fourth year; student teach; graduate; begin teaching. Your goal should be something you are willing to work hard for, not something you just "want." It should not be something dangerous to yourself or others, such as stealing forty cars by next week or taking drugs so you do not have to face your problems. It does not have to involve getting more education. Your goal may be to get a job so you can support your family, or it might be as simple as learning to take better care of your children. Set goals one at a time, so you can give all your attention to that *one*, and then go step by step until you reach it. (Go around the group and ask each member what goal he or she wants most to reach, then ask what the first few steps would be to reach that goal and if he or she is willing to do what it takes to reach it.) (Time: 15 minutes.)

• Do the relaxation exercise. Give instructions as follows (Time: 10 minutes):

> Now we are going to do a relaxation exercise. Some of you may not be familiar with this, but it helps relieve stress and puts a mini-vacation into your day. It is a good way to relax before going to sleep or anytime you feel

stressed. Everyone get as comfortable as possible before we start. (You may want to darken the room somewhat.)

Close your eyes and breathe in . . . and out . . . gently through your nose or mouth; allow yourself to become more and more relaxed. As you gently breathe in . . . and . . . out, your feet become relaxed (pause), your legs become relaxed (pause), your abdomen becomes relaxed (pause), your back and shoulders become relaxed (pause), and your arms and hands become relaxed (pause). And as you continue to breathe in . . . and . . . out, gently and quietly, your head becomes relaxed and your mind floats free. You find yourself floating away from this room to a place where you feel happy and free. It may be a place in nature, a place you have visited on vacation, or anywhere where you feel good about yourself. When you get there, just enjoy being there. Enjoy the warmth of the sun . . . and breathe it into yourself. Feel the warmth of the sun and feel filled with love. Now see yourself as perfect exactly the way you are . . . as a friend (pause) . . . with your family (pause) . . . with yourself. See yourself at ease with something that you enjoy doing, whether it is listening to music, dancing, singing, talking with friends, caring for your family, or being alone. Just experience the joy of being you (pause). Continue to feel the warmth of the sun and to breathe in a feeling of peace and well-being while we pause here for a while (pause 1-2 minutes). Now let yourself begin to come back. Bring this feeling of well-being with you, and carry it with you throughout the day. I will count to three. Open your eyes at the count of three. One . . . two . . . three. (Adapted from *Spinning Inward*, by Maureen Murdock, Shambhala Publishers, 1987.)

• Distribute evaluation forms; have pencils available. Names are optional. Collect them facedown on one of the tables. (Time: 5 minutes.)

• Hold the Pretty Prize drawing. Be sure all group members are entered. The same person cannot win two weeks in succession. (Time: 5 minutes.)

• Do the Car Wash exercise if time allows.

Chapter 17

Week Fifteen: Celebration

Goals for the Week Are:

1. To celebrate finishing several or all weeks, if this is a close-
   ended course
2. To learn to work and get along with others through games and
   activities

Materials Needed:

A Participant Handbook for each group member
Pens, felt-tip markers, and notebook or paper for sign-in
Name tags
Pencils for participants
Any materials needed for a chosen craft, talent show, fashion
   show, etc.
"Outburst," "Charades," "Win, Lose, or Draw," or any other
   group game
Large package of uncooked spaghetti
Large package of small, soft gumdrops
Tape player and tape of energizing music
Collection of varied objects, more than members in the group
   (See instructions for "Get Acquainted Objects" if that is chosen
   as an activity.)
Chalkboard, flip chart, or large pad of drawing paper
Pretty Prize(s)

Celebration week can finish the LAMS series if it has been a close-ended group or can be used as a time to celebrate life by learning to have fun and get along with others. Food should be more festive than usual with dessert included. An upcoming holiday could serve as a theme for the week. The group participants may want to plan the activities, which might be a fashion show, talent show, games, puppet show, an invited guest, or a craft project. If they do not wish to do this, the facilitator should follow the activities indicated.

Begin, as always, by reading the Affirmation for the week aloud, in unison; group members should read from their handbooks. Then read the information about the LAMS program aloud to everyone.

The game, "Geography," is played next. This week it is just for "fun," not for any other purpose. Instructions are in the following material.

Activities for the day may vary. Team games have been very popular with past groups. Game-playing can cause bickering and arguments, but peer pressure usually is enough to end any problems. Games are seldom played in many of the participants' homes, even with their children. Some group members never do anything "just for fun" and need to learn that it is okay for them to do so; life needs to be *lived*, not just *endured*.

Several activities have been tried during this session. The "Outburst" game has been very successful, as it is easy to play in a large group and is not as difficult a game as "Trivial Pursuit." Remember that many group members have low educational levels and often have not read extensively. Things they pick up from daily life or from TV are included in "Outburst."

The food for break should be more festive today. Cake and ice cream, or other celebratory food, should be included to make this week special. Group members could plan the menu and even have a "pot-luck" meal, but be sure leaders bring basics in case someone forgets or cannot afford what they volunteered to bring.

If certificates from the Expanded Nutrition Program are to be given at this session that can be included now. If this has been a close-ended session, and all of the group members will be graduating, conduct a ceremony and take pictures, if desired.

The participants may opt to continue playing games after the break, or the leader may want to use one of the listed activities, such as "Get-Acquainted Objects" or "Spaghetti Structures." The spaghetti exercise is particularly helpful, as LAMS group members often have problems relating to others and may be quite isolated. They often have problems at work because they cannot get along with their co-workers or the customers. The constructions from spaghetti and gumdrops illustrate how important it is to work as a team. Getting something built can be frustrating but fun as well. Some of the constructions are complex and very innovative. It is amazing that they have been built with no conversation and no original known goal.

Conclude the session with evaluations, the Pretty Prize drawing, and the Car Wash exercise.

Remember to give each graduate a Graduation Questionnaire to complete. These are very helpful in learning how useful the graduates found LAMS to be and if it has helped them to change their lives. If they were referred by someone else, ask that person to complete the Post-LAMS Questionnaire so it can be compared with the results noted by the participants.

If this has been a close-ended program, return to Week One next time with a new group. If it is an ongoing program, proceed with the present members to Week One and add new ones as they are referred. Participants can successfully start at any point in the program and continue until they reach the week preceding the week they began, and then graduate. Each week stands alone, and the material can be presented in any order, as long as the whole LAMS program is completed.

WEEK FIFTEEN: CELEBRATION

• Register all new members and give each a Participant Handbook and Pre-LAMS Questionnaire to be completed and handed in at the end of the session.

• Introduce the facilitator(s), give a brief description of the LAMS program, and discuss housekeeping issues. (Time: 5 minutes.)

• Read the Affirmation aloud, in unison; participants should read from their handbooks. (Time: 5 minutes.)

> I am a good person.
> I am a happy person.
> I can do anything I set my mind to, if I really work hard.
> There are some things I cannot change; I will learn
>   to accept these things.
> I have a right to enjoy myself and others around me,
>   to laugh and play.

• The facilitator should read the following aloud:

> You learn many things in LAMS. If you are at or near completion of the course, you will remember many of the lessons and hopefully are practicing them. If you have just begun to attend, you have many sessions ahead of you that will give you a blueprint for changing your life. Positive affirmations, or things that make you feel good about yourself, should become a part of your thinking every day. What you think determines how you feel. Learning to make choices, set goals, and get along with others are all important parts of the LAMS program. You have learned, or will learn, that what you heard as a child is not necessarily true today and, in fact, may not have been true then. Education, good health, sensible shopping, and proper nutrition are all keys to living the kind of life you want to live. Through all of these teachings, the LAMS program should enable you to be in control of your own life.
>
> Nobody can *make* you change, but LAMS can show you *how* to change, if you really want to. I hope you will decide to live your life by choice, not by chance.

• Play the warm-up game, "Geography," from *Action Speaks Louder*, by Remocker and Storch. The first person to play says the name of a place (New York). The next person gives another geographical name that begins with the last letter of the previous one (Kansas), continuing around the group. Places can be towns, cities, states, countries, or even continents. Clues can be given if someone cannot think of a name. (Time: 10 minutes.)

• Activities for this week can be planned by the group participants in advance or by the leader. Possibilities could be a talent show, fashion show (maybe of resale or donated clothing), games, puppet show, an invited guest, or a craft project. (Time: 40 minutes.)

Playing games can help group members learn to get along with others and work as a team. One game that is very successful with a group is "Outburst," available in most toy or department stores. Players call out possible answers in specified categories and get points for each answer that matches one of the ten on the game card (for example, "Things found in a woman's purse" or "Brands of candy bars"). Do not use the game board. Either a facilitator or group member should be timekeeper and keep score on the score-board provided with the game. Divide the group into two teams, alternating asking questions from the game cards. Eliminate cards with topics that seem too difficult for the group to answer readily.

Other possible games are "Charades," and "Win, Lose, or Draw," or any others designed for group play. Games intended for smaller groups of players can be played with teams and without using the game board.

• Announce time for a break and food. Food today should be more festive than usual. Party foods such as cake and ice cream might be added, or the group may decide to have a pot-luck dinner with everyone bringing something. (Let group members bring extras, but provide the basics in case someone forgets or does not have enough money to fix something.) (Time: 30 minutes.)

• If you have included the Department of Agriculture Expanded Nutrition Program in your curriculum, have their representative award certificates of completion at this time. (Time: 5 minutes.)

• Continue games if the group wishes to continue, or the facilitator may decide to do the "Get-Acquainted Objects" exercise instead. This is an exercise that builds acceptance and teamwork. Present a collection of varied objects, a larger number than there are participants. Suggested objects are shells, puppets, tools, toys, or office supplies. These can be things around the office or group setting, not necessarily things brought in. Each group member should choose an item they like. They then tell about themselves through the item they chose. They might explain how they are alike or different from their chosen object or how it relates to their personality or hobbies. They are to be as creative as possible. (Time: 20 minutes.)

• Do the "Spaghetti Structures" exercise. The facilitator will need a large package of uncooked spaghetti, a large package of small, soft gumdrops, and a tape player and tape of energizing music. Divide the group members into small groups of up to six persons. Divide the spaghetti and gumdrops equally among the groups. Give the following instructions.

1. Starting now, you may not talk or communicate with words.
2. You are to build a "something" using the materials you were given.
3. You must decide how and what you will do without talking or writing notes.
4. After you finish, you may talk to pick a name for your structure.

We will then discuss what each team built and how they did it.
Turn on the tape of music while they work.
After all the structures are finished, ask the following questions:

How did you decide who was the leader? . . . How were decisions made? . . . Did you work together to make something, or did each of you try to make what *you* wanted to make? . . . Did everyone in the group help with the building? . . . Did you get angry or frustrated because the spaghetti broke easily? . . . How did you handle that if you did? . . . Do you feel good about how you helped or what you did while you were working together? . . . Original source of this exercise was the Multi-State HIV Project for High Risk Youth at the University of Utah. (Time: 25 minutes.)

• Distribute evaluation forms; have pencils available. Names are optional. Collect them facedown on one of the tables. (Time: 5 minutes.)

• Hold the Pretty Prize drawing. Be sure all group members are entered. The same person cannot win two weeks in succession. (Time: 5 minutes.)

• Do the Car Wash exercise if time allows.

Appendix

The Role of Psychoeducational Groups in Enhancing Personal Relationships and Social Networks: Final Report

Marianne Berry

OBJECTIVES

This study examined the use and effectiveness of psychoeducational support groups in the local, public child welfare agency in achieving positive case outcomes and in increasing social relationship skills and social networks. *Learning About Myself (LAMS)* is a psychoeducational group for mothers, focusing on self-esteem and relationship skills.

REVIEW OF THE LITERATURE

This study seeks to focus on the role of psychoeducational support groups in achieving positive outcomes for children and families served by public child welfare agencies. Public child welfare agencies are charged with the prevention and treatment of child maltreatment, with the priority of preserving families while keeping children safe (Barth and Berry, 1994). Achieving such a complex objective requires a sound knowledge base of risks associated with child abuse

This research was supported by a National Child Welfare Fellowship from the U.S. Children's Bureau to the author. The author thanks Nancy Dickinson, Sherrill Clark, and the staff of the California Social Work Education Center at the University of California for their supervision and guidance during this fellowship. The author is also grateful to her fellow fellows for their input and guidance during this research effort. Special thanks to Verna Rickard with the Texas Department of Protective and Regulatory Services for her support of this project. Thanks also to Scottye Cash, doctoral student in the UTA School of Social Work, for data entry, management, and analysis and assistance with the literature.

and neglect, the resources associated with family well-being, and a strong practice base of the techniques and programs that are effective in a variety of circumstances, cultures, and populations.

Certainly, parents and families need to possess particular skills and resources in order to sustain and nurture their members. Child abuse and neglect are related to poor parenting skills, parental depression, family stress, economic hardship, and other characteristics and conditions (Garbarino and Gilliam, 1980; McDonald and Marks, 1991). Many studies have also identified social isolation as a key correlate of child maltreatment (Belle, 1982; Brunk, Henggeler, and Whelan, 1987; Crittenden, 1985; Darmstadt, 1990; Leifer, Shapiro, and Kassem, 1993; Strauss, 1980; Zuravin and Greif, 1989).

On the other hand, not all families have the same combination or configuration of risks and service needs. Evaluations of families and services must provide information on the match of services to needs (Berry, 1992). An important, but often neglected, element of program evaluation in child welfare and family preservation services is the documentation of the specific goals each family or client has. Services provided are intended to differ from family to family and be individualized to the strengths and needs of the family (based on a risk and strengths assessment). It is important, therefore, to examine services and goals in order to assess the relevance of service provision to client goals.

Many have posited that, without attention to the social relationship needs and skills of parents, advice and training concerning parenting or other family care strategies will not be effective or lasting (Cochran, 1991; Lovell, Reid, and Richey, 1991; Miller and Whittaker, 1988; Whittaker and Tracy, 1988). Indeed, Patterson, Chamberlain, and Reid (1982) have found that parent training "enhanced" by attention to relationship skills results in bigger and more durable gains in parenting skills. Griest and colleagues (1982) have also found "enhanced" parent training to produce improvement in parenting, longer lasting effects, and greater generalizability to other skills.

Lovell and colleagues (1991) evaluated a program to enhance socially supportive networks for low-income abusive mothers. The program followed an agency-based parenting group that was a form of "enhanced" parenting education, which taught and rehearsed skills basic to friendship and self-assertion in relationships. The program was developed in reaction to the finding that the parenting group alone, while providing opportunities for friendship and ongoing relationships, did not result in increases in social networks over time. An evaluation of the enhanced social-support training found significant increases in social network size as well as improved quality and quantity of social interactions. Associated reductions in child maltreatment were not addressed.

Cochran's (1991) study of the Family Matters program in New York found that a community-based program for 160 families with three-year-olds was successful in enlarging social networks, as compared to a control group who did not receive the program. Participation in the program was associated with greater linkages to supports and higher perceptions of self as parent for both unmarried and married mothers. However, there were key cultural differences, which were corroborated by other research highlighting differences in social support across cultures (Timberlake and Chipungu, 1992). For white mothers, growth largely took place with nonrelated social network members, and this growth was associated with enhanced parental identity and the child's improved performance in school. The majority of increases in the social network were confined to relatives for black mothers, however. Among black, unmarried mothers, growth in the social network of relatives was associated with increases in parent-child activities, while growth in the social network of nonrelatives was associated with the child's improved academic performance.

Despite the caveat that families served by public child welfare agencies are poor candidates for group attendance and participation (Polansky, Ammons, and Gaudin, 1985; Polansky et al., 1981), the Tarrant County agency has developed and provided these groups over a number of years and enjoys high participation rates. To date, however, there had been no concerted evaluation conducted by an independent researcher.

LEARNING ABOUT MYSELF

Method

Procedure

The Learning About Myself psychoeducational support group meets weekly at the public child protective services agency for twelve weeks. This is a group for both women and men, attended primarily by women, who are taught to be more assertive, make better choices, and improve their self-esteem. Much of the group activities include hands-on activities such as games, crafts, and role-plays. Positive affirmations are used weekly, including a "Pretty Prize" awarded each week to a group member. Over the twelve weeks of the course, the following twelve topics are emphasized and explored: my self, my attitude, my relationships, my appearance, my time for myself, my friends, my education, my health, my family, my finances, my home, and my goals, then a celebration. Each week's content stands alone to minimize the negative effects of absences. Clients are free to attend on an open-ended basis, attending sessions they may have missed in the past. Transportation and child care are provided to group members.

Much of the curriculum emphasizes taking charge of one's life and recognizing choices where clients may see none. The presentation of many topics is nurturing and fun, through playing games, making crafts, and so on. For example, participants make hair bows together, and many times this is the first time they have made something attractive and functional. During "budgeting" week, participants play "The Price is Right" with paired generic and brand-name products, and the winners take the products home.

Sample

The sample for this study consisted of all mothers who attended the Learning About Myself psychoeducational support group in either 1994 or 1995, and who had completed both an entry questionnaire and a graduation questionnaire, and for whom a caseworker had also completed graduation questionnaires concerning the needs and progress of the client. This sampling frame is very conservative, eliminating those clients for whom there were any missing questionnaires out of the three mentioned above, and resulted in a sample of nineteen mothers.

Design

This evaluation utilized a one-group posttest only design. Although clients and their caseworkers filled out a questionnaire upon entry and at case closure, the measures at posttest do not match those at intake and thus, do not provide any measures of change from pretest to posttest. Therefore, only posttest measures provide any indication of program effects or rather, perceptions of effects.

Measures

The Texas Department of Protective and Regulatory Services has preexisting instruments for each support group it offers. This study used these preexisting measures in the evaluation of this group and subsequently modified these instruments as a recommendation at the end of the study.

The preexisting instruments (for LAMS) consisted of three questionnaires. The client filled out a questionnaire at intake and another questionnaire at graduation from the group. Similarly, the client's caseworker filled out a questionnaire after the client's graduation from the group.

The intake questionnaires asked the client about the following: her childhood experiences and beliefs, goals for herself and her family, and beliefs about her self (self-efficacy, appearance, social support and friendships, etc.). Most of these were in the form of open-ended questions to which the client could write a brief response. These written responses generated coded categories of responses, designed by the researcher.

The graduation questionnaires asked about the client's and/or caseworker's perceptions of the usefulness or effectiveness of the group, both globally and in specific terms, and the client's current perceptions of self-efficacy, appearance, social support and friendships, and so on.

Results

Client Characteristics

Nineteen mothers are included in this sample. Almost 50 percent were born prior to 1970 (were at least twenty-seven years old), but 25 percent were between the ages of eighteen and twenty-seven (see Table 1). Most lived in poverty, with almost 50 percent reporting an annual income under $9,000. The vast majority of group members

TABLE 1. Learning About Myself—Client Characteristics and Presenting Problems

Characteristic	Respondents (n=19)
Client's birth year	
1955 to 1959	11 %
1960 to 1969	37
1970 to 1979	26
Unknown	26
Annual family income	
Under $9,000	48 %
$9,000 to $17,999	21
$18,000 or over	5
Unknown	26
Number of children	
One	31 %
Two	53
Three	8
Four	8
Marital status	
Married	47 %
Single	21
Separated	11
Divorced	11
Unknown	10
Client's ethnicity	
Caucasian	58 %
African American	16
Hispanic	16
Unknown	10
Type(s) of child maltreatment currently reported*	
Physical abuse	26 %
Physical neglect	26
Medical neglect	16
Neglectful supervision	11
Sexual abuse	5
Unknown	26

*Column may total more than 100% due to multiple responses.

had either one (31 percent) or two (53 percent) children. Almost 50 percent were married, and another 43 percent were classified as single, though they may have once been married. They often were living with someone or had been in several relationships. Over half of the group members were Caucasian (58 percent), with equal percentage of African-American (16 percent) and Hispanic (16 percent) group members.

There was variation in the types of child abuse for which these women were receiving child protective services, with some form of child neglect most prevalent. About 25 percent of the mothers had been reported for physical neglect, 16 percent for medical neglect, and 11 percent for neglectful supervision of their child(ren). Another 25 percent had been reported for physical abuse of their child(ren). The type of abuse reported was unknown for about 25 percent of these respondents.

Client Background and Past Experiences

Upon entering the Learning About Myself group, members were asked to complete a two-page questionnaire asking them, in open-ended fashion, about their childhood and their hopes and dreams. Many of these women had been abused in childhood (see Table 2). About half had been either emotionally abused (53 percent) and/or neglected (47 percent), and many had experienced physical abuse (32 percent), incest (21 percent), and/or sexual abuse by a nonrelative (21 percent). About one-third of group members had also experienced some form of abuse in adulthood.

Mothers were also asked what they, as children, had wanted to be when they grew up. Answers varied and displayed the normal range of career goals for young women (see Table 2), including nurse, doctor, mother, and teacher. When asked "What did you never have as a child that you wanted?", responses also varied, with one-third mentioning some material goods, such as toys.

Family members play influential roles in the lives of group members. When asked who had changed their lives the most, over half of respondents named either their spouse/partner (32 percent) or their children (21 percent). Friends were named as most influential by only 11 percent of group members (see Table 2).

TABLE 2. Learning About Myself—Childhood and Past Experiences

Characteristic	Respondents (n=19)
Experienced the following in childhood*	
Emotional abuse	53 %
Neglect	47
Physical abuse	32
Incest	21
Sexual abuse by a nonrelative	21
Experienced the following in adulthood*	
Spousal abuse	37 %
Sexual abuse by a nonrelative	32
What did you want to be when you grew up?*	
Nurse	21 %
Doctor	16
Mother	16
Teacher	16
Beautician	11
Airline Stewardess	5
Computer Technician	5
Fireman	5
Musician	5
Writer	5
Other	15
What did you never have as a child that you wanted?*	
Toys/material things	32 %
Nothing	22
Love	16
Support	11
A childhood	5
A good home	5
A lot of things	5
A sister	5
Freedom	5
My own room	5
Privacy	5
To be normal	5
Person who has changed your life the most	
Partner/spouse	32 %
Children	21
No one	15
Parents	11
Friend/neighbor	11
Spiritual person	5
Other relative	5

*Column may total more than 100% due to multiple responses.

Client Beliefs and Coping Strategies

About 25 percent of the group members reported feeling happy about their life. More were ambivalent (32 percent), and many were angry (21 percent) or sad (11 percent). When asked what members did to feel better or to have fun, responses varied across personal and social activities (see Table 3).

Group members were asked what they liked most and disliked most about themselves. Twenty-five percent of the mothers said they liked nothing about themselves, while another quarter (26 percent) were most proud of their children and family (see Table 3). Many also felt good about the way they treat others (21 percent). Comments about personal dislikes centered primarily around personality characteristics (42 percent) and appearance (26 percent), rather than more instrumental abilities.

Client Goals

Several questions on the intake questionnaire asked about client goals (see Table 4). When asked about personal goals, group members were somewhat vague and/or gloomy in their responses. When asked how they would most like to change their lives, one-fifth (21 percent) said they would like to change their outlook, and another 16 percent could not identify a primary goal regarding changing their lives. Two respondents (11 percent) named the return of their children from foster care as their primary goal. (Not many of their children were out of the home).

More specific questions asked about activities group members would like to pursue (see Table 4). Travel was the activity mentioned most by members (26 percent) when asked what they had always wanted to do but had never done. Another fifth (21 percent) named a career choice, and an additional 16 percent mentioned more education.

Similarly, when asked what they wanted most for their children (see Table 4), many named an education (21 percent). Additional answers varied, but many women named independence (15 percent), happiness (11 percent), and a productive/successful or responsible life (11 percent). Similarly, when group members were asked about

TABLE 3. Learning About Myself—Client Beliefs and Coping Strategies

Characteristic	Respondents (n=19)
How do you feel about your life?	
Ambivalent	32 %
Happy	26
Angry	21
Sad	11
Life happens	5
Life is hard	5
What do you do to feel better about yourself?*	
Take care of myself	26 %
Make personal changes	16
Read	16
Be with others	11
Buy things	11
Go out	11
Cook	5
Exercise	5
Listen to music	5
Nothing	5
Pray	5
What do you do for fun?*	
Be outside	32 %
Spend time together with family	26
Listen to music	21
Go to movies	16
Play sports	16
Watch television	16
Go shopping	11
Read	5
What do you like most about yourself?	
Children and family	26 %
Nothing	21
The way I treat others	21
Personality	11
Specific body feature	11
Confidence	5
The way I treat myself	5
What do you dislike the most about yourself?	
Personality characteristics	42 %
Weight/appearance	26
Dependency	11
Education and/or job skills	11
Everything	5
Unable to provide for children	5

*Column may total more than 100% due to multiple responses.

TABLE 4. Learning About Myself—Client Goals

Characteristic	Respondents (n=19)
How would you most like to change your life?	
Outlook	21 %
Nothing	16
Children returned	11
Education	11
Financial security	11
Accomplish something	11
Car	5
Family change	5
Job change	5
Living situation	5
Relationship	5
What have you always wanted to do that you have never done?	
Travel	26 %
Career choice	21
Education	16
Adventure	11
Nothing	11
Drive a new car	5
Relationship	5
Spend money freely	5
What is the one thing you want most for your children?	
Education	21 %
Be independent	15
Be happy	11
Be productive/successful/responsible	11
Have a better life	11
Have a good career	11
Be healthy	5
Be loving and respectful	5
Have everything they need	5
Love without being afraid	5
What would you want your life to be like five years from now?*	
Own my own home	32 %
Have a better family life	21
Be happy	16
Be independent	16
Better than now	16
Financial security	16
Have a new job	16
Be better educated	5
Own/purchase a new car	5

Characteristic	Respondents (n=19)
What one thing have you always wanted to know about or learn to do?	
Nothing	31 %
Musical instrument	16
Computers/technology	11
Crafts/home improvement	11
Medicine	11
Cars	11
Education	5
Law	5
Parenting	5
What would you most like to change about your looks?	
Nothing	37 %
Shape/weight	37
Hair	11
Demeanor	5
Everything	5
Face	5
Of all the things you could buy, what do you want most that there is a real chance you could get?*	
Housing	37 %
Car	26
Clothes	26
Appliances	16
Happiness	5
Self-improvement	5
Things for children	5
What would you most like to have in your house that you don't have right now?	
Furniture	31 %
Appliances	21
Electronics	16
Everything	11
My children	11
Extra bedroom	5
Peace	5

*Column may total more than 100% due to multiple responses.

their own goals for themselves five years from now, many mentioned economic stability or self-sufficiency—home ownership (32 percent), financial security (16 percent), a new job (16 percent), and a new car (5 percent). These answers are particularly interesting, given their discrepancy from mothers' criticisms of themselves (see Table 3) centering around features of personality and appearance.

Group members were also asked what one thing they have always wanted to know about or do, and many (31 percent) said nothing (see Table 4). Answers varied a great deal, with some respondents wanting to learn a musical instrument and others wanting to learn about computers. When asked what about their looks they would like to change, many group members again said nothing (37 percent), although another 37 percent would like to change their shape or weight.

Two questions asked about clients' material wants and the responses belied the significant issues of housing and material deprivation among child protective services clients (see Table 4). When asked "Of all the things you could buy, what do you want most that there is a real chance you could get?", group members often named housing (37 percent), a car (26 percent), clothing (26 percent), and appliances (16 percent). Also, when asked "What would you most like to have in your house that you don't have right now?", group members most often mentioned furniture (31 percent), appliances (21 percent), and electronics (16 percent), although two respondents said "my children" (11 percent).

*Client and Caseworker Perceptions of Group Effects
at Graduation*

Both the client and caseworker ratings of the effects of the Learning About Myself groups are uniformly positive and in close agreement, with caseworkers slightly less positive about the effects of the group for their clients (see Table 5). Almost all clients agreed that they had (1) learned new ways to solve problems or make decisions, (2) become more assertive, and (3) improved in parenting skills. Somewhat lower numbers of caseworkers saw these same effects but still in relatively high proportions. There was a significant difference in age between those mothers about whom caseworkers reported an improvement in parenting skills, with those improving being younger on average (25 years old) than those not improving (33 years old). Similarly, those mothers about whom caseworkers reported being more assertive were younger on average (26 years old) than were those mothers for whom caseworkers saw no difference in assertiveness (32 years old).

TABLE 5. Learning About Myself—Client Goals

Characteristic	Group Members	Case- workers* (n=19)
Did the client learn new ways to solve problems or make decisions?	95 %	77 %
Did the client become more assertive?	95	72
Did the client's parenting skills improve?	90	60
Did the client's appearance improve?	74	65
Do you (client) believe that individuals who used to feel helpless can learn to be more powerful?	100	
Do you (client) feel that you have choices and that life does not just "happen" to you?	90	
Have you (client) done anything that you used to be afraid of?	26	
Is LAMS effective?		100
Have you (caseworker) seen any indications that your client's self-esteem has increased?		89
Do you (caseworker) think that your client's attendance will contribute to earlier case closure?		88
Have your client's children improved in appearance?		53
Is your client more independent?		44
Social Networks and Social Isolation		
Have you (client) made new friends since becoming a LAMS member?	100	
Average number of new friends	5	
Have you (client) talked on the phone or visited other LAMS members between sessions?	21	
Does your client seek help from others more now?		83
Is your client as socially isolated?		18

*Sample size of caseworkers reflects caseworker responses, rather than the number of caseworkers referring clients to LAMS.

Fewer group members felt that their appearance had improved over the course of group attendance, although their caseworkers were in close agreement about improvements in appearance. All women who had experienced spousal abuse said their appearance had improved as a function of attending LAMS, as compared to approximately 58 percent of those who had not experienced spousal abuse.

Group members were also asked about issues of empowerment and assertiveness. One hundred percent of clients said that they believed that individuals who used to feel helpless can learn to be more powerful (see Table 5), and 90 percent said that they now feel that they have choices and that life does not "just happen." Over a quarter of group members had tried something they used to be afraid of while attending Learning About Myself.

Caseworkers also felt that Learning About Myself is an effective experience for their clients (see Table 5). Many saw indications of improvements in self-esteem (89 percent), improvements in the children's appearance (53 percent), and greater independence (44 percent). Almost all caseworkers felt that attendance at LAMS would contribute to an earlier closure of the client's child protective services case.

Finally, regarding issues of social isolation and enhancements to social networks, clients were asked if they had made new friends since attending Learning About Myself (see Table 5). All clients said they had increased their social supports (100 percent), with an average of five new friends per client. One-fifth of group members had talked on the phone or visited another LAMS member between group sessions. Talking on the phone was significantly more likely among divorced and single women than among married women. Caseworkers also felt that clients had increased their ability to seek help as a result of attending LAMS (83 percent), and only 18 percent felt that their client was as socially isolated as when they had begun attending Learning About Myself.

Clients were asked in specific terms about the most effective elements of the Learning About Myself group experience (see Table 6). Group members could answer as many items as applied. While the most commonly mentioned element concerned learning how to make choices (90 percent), experiencing warm relationships within the group was mentioned by 79 percent of members as a helpful element of

LAMS. Equally helpful were learning how to be assertive and learning how to identify and accept feelings. A few group members said that they wished they had learned more about relationships (16 percent).

Over half of all group members (58 percent) were attending some other counseling or class while attending Learning About Myself. Many of the members attended parenting classes (26 percent), ROAR assertiveness group for abused women (11 percent), or individual psychological counseling (11 percent). All women who had experienced spousal abuse had also attended some other form of counseling while attending LAMS, as compared to the approximately 33 percent of those not experiencing spousal abuse.

A full two-thirds of the clients attending LAMS (68 percent) experienced a successful closure of their child protective services case (see Table 6). Another 10 percent of clients were referred from intensive family preservation services to some other, less intensive service unit or agency. A full 22 percent of cases, however, were not closed at the end of data collection, or the outcome of the case was unknown. Outcomes did not differ across types of abuse reported.

Discussion

Learning About Myself is aimed at low-income women with low self-esteem. The nineteen participants in the LAMS groups showed many indications of poverty and material deprivations, low self-esteem, and social isolation at entry into the group. At the closure of the group, however, both client and caseworker ratings of the effects of the group are uniformly positive. Almost all clients agreed that they had learned new ways to solve problems, become more assertive, and improved in parenting skills. All clients said they had made new friends, some of whom were LAMS members but not all. Learning About Myself, therefore, appears to contribute to improvements in these women's lives, particularly in their relationship skills and problem-solving skills.

It is important to note the contribution of the pretest questionnaires to the evaluation but, more important, to the substance of the group. Questions inquiring about clients' hopes and dreams rather than their immediate needs and methods of compliance with caseworker demands probably helped to engage clients in the process of the group and were integrated and completely congruent with the

TABLE 6. Learning About Myself—Client Perceptions of Group Effectiveness

Characteristic	Respondents (n=19)
What was the most helpful to you about LAMS?*	
Learning how to make choices that can change my life	90 %
Experiencing warm relationships within the group	79
Learning how to be assertive, not passive or aggres- sive	79
Learning how to identify and accept my feelings	79
Learning how my past experiences affect the present	74
Other	11
I wish we had learned more about:	
Relationships	16 %
My self	11
Each other	5
Nothing	68
Attended additional and concurrent counseling	58 %
Parenting classes	26
ROAR-Assertiveness	11
Individual counseling	11
Anger control	5
Mental health/mental retardation classes	5
Case outcome	
Case successfully closed	68 %
Case referred to other, less intensive unit	5
Case referred to contract services (less intensive)	5
Outcome unknown/case not closed	22

*Column may total more than 100% due to multiple responses.

substance of the group. For many clients, this was the first time in a service setting that they were asked about themselves in a positive manner and the first time that their own personal goals were inquired about and respected.

Recommendations

Considering the uniformly high ratings given the Learning About Myself group by both participants and caseworkers, lengthy recommendations for improvement of the group are not warranted. Anecdotal evidence suggests that the originator and author of the LAMS curriculum, Verna Rickard, is to be credited with much of the success of Learning About Myself. Ms. Rickard is noted by many to be highly nurturing, clear, and creative, and her contributions to the success of LAMS are substantial.

Therefore, the effective replication of Learning About Myself by others is dependent upon clear information about the groups. This training manual on the group will be extremely important to replication efforts. This manual contains curriculum content and exercises, including worksheets and questions, and it is recommended that replication efforts adhere closely to this successful curriculum.

It is this author's recommendation also that the qualitative questionnaires at pretest that ask about the clients' childhood experiences and future hopes and dreams be retained in any replication. As mentioned above, these questionnaires appear to be integral to group curriculum, client engagement, and evaluation efforts.

If additional measures were to be added to an evaluation of Learning About Myself in the future, I suggest that clear information on client demographic characteristics and presenting problems be gathered at pretest, and that a follow-up questionnaire or phone call be administered at six months after treatment to assess the longevity of effects.

References for Professionals

Barth, Richard P., and Marianne Berry (1994). Implications of research on the welfare of children under permanency planning. In Richard Barth, Jill D. Berrick, and Neil Gilbert (Eds.), *Child Welfare Research Review.* New York: Columbia University Press.

Belle, Deborah (1982). Social ties and social support. In Deborah Belle (Ed.), *Lives In Stress: Women and Depression.* Beverly Hills, CA: Sage Publications.

Berry, Marianne (1988). A review of parent training programs in child welfare. *Social Service Review* 62 (2): 302-323.

Berry, Marianne (1992). An evaluation of family preservation services: Fitting agency services to family needs. *Social Work* 37: 314-321.

Breines, Wini, and Linda Gordon (1983). The new scholarship on family violence. *Signs: Journal of Women in Culture and Society* 8: 490-531.

Brunk, M., Scott W. Henggeler, and J.P. Whelan (1987). Comparison of multisystemic therapy and parent training in the brief treatment of child abuse and neglect. *Journal of Consulting and Clinical Psychology* 55: 171-178.

Canfield, Jack, and Harold C. Wells (1976). *100 Ways to Enhance Self-Concept in the Classroom: A Handbook for Teachers and Parents.* Upper Saddle River, NJ: Prentice Hall.

Cochran, Moncreif (1991). Personal social networks as a focus of support. *Prevention in Human Services* 9: 45-67.

Cohn, Anne Harris, and Deborah Daro (1987). Is treatment too late: What ten years of evaluative research tell us. *Child Abuse and Neglect* 11: 433-442.

Crittenden, Patricia (1985). Social networks, quality of child rearing, and child development. *Child Development* 56: 1299-1313.

Darmstadt, G. (1990). Community-based child abuse prevention. *Social Work* 35: 487-493.

Dumas, Jean E. (1986). Parental perception and treatment outcome in families of aggressive children: A causal model. *Behavior Therapy* 17: 420-432.

Fluegelman, Andrew (1976). *The New Games Book.* Berkeley, CA: Headlands Press.

Forehand, Rex L., and R.J. McMahon (1981). *Helping the Non-Compliant Child: A Clinician's Guide to Parent Training.* New York: Guilford.

Gaines, Richard, Alice Sandgrund, Arthur H. Green, and Ernest Power (1978). Etiological factors in child maltreatment: A multivariate study of abusing, neglecting, and normal mothers. *Journal of Abnormal Psychology* 87: 531-540.

Garbarino, James (1976). A preliminary study of some ecological correlates of child abuse: The impact of socioeconomic stress on mothers. *Child Development* 47: 178-185.

Garbarino, James (1977). The human ecology of child maltreatment: A conceptual model for research. *Journal of Marriage and the Family* 39: 721-735.

Garbarino, James, and G. Gilliam (1980). *Understanding Abusive Families.* Lexington, MA: Lexington Books.

Gick Publishing (1990). *Hairbows for Kids.* Irvine, CA.

Griest, Douglas L., and Rex Forehand (1982). How can I get any parent training done with all these other problems going on? The role of family variables in child behavior therapy. *Child and Family Behavior Therapy* 4: 73-80.

Griest, Douglas L., Rex Forehand, Thomas Rogers, J. Breiner, William Furey, and Cheryl A. Williams (1982). Effects of parent enhancement therapy on the treatment outcome and generalization of a parent training program. *Behavior Research and Therapy* 20: 429-436.

Helmstetter, Saul (1989). *Choices.* New York: Pocket Books.

Johnson, Will, and Jill L'Esperance (1984). Predicting the recurrence of child abuse. *Social Work Research and Abstracts* 20: 21-31.

Leifer, M., J.P. Shapiro, and L. Kassem (1993). The impact of maternal history and behavior upon foster placement and adjustment in sexually abused girls. *Child Abuse and Neglect* 17: 755-766.

Lovell, Madeline L., Kathy Reid, and Cheryl A. Richey (1991). Social support training for abusive mothers. In James A. Garland (Ed.), *Group Work Reaching Out: People, Places and Power.* Binghamton, NY: The Haworth Press, Inc..

Lovell, Madeline L., Kathy Reid, and Cheryl A. Richey (1992). Social support training for abusive mothers. In James A. Garland (Ed.), *Group Work Reaching Out: People, Places and Power.* Binghamton, NY: The Haworth Press, Inc..

McClelland, David (1973). Testing for competence rather than intelligence. *American Psychologist* 28: 1-14.

McDonald, Thomas and Jill Marks (1991). A review of risk factors assessed in child protective services. *Social Service Review* 65: 112-132.

Miller, J.L., and James K. Whittaker (1988). Social services and support: Blended programs for families at risk of child maltreatment. *Child Welfare* 67: 161-174.

Murdock, Maureen (1987). *Spinning Inward.* Boston, MA: Shambhala.

Parke, R., and C.W. Collmer (1975). Child abuse: An interdisciplinary analysis. In Eileen Mavis Hetherington (Ed.), *Review of Child Developmental Research.* Chicago, IL: University of Chicago Press.

Patterson, Gerald R. (1980). Mothers: The unacknowledged victims. *Monographs of The Society for Research in Child Development* 45 (5): 1-64.

Patterson, Gerald R. (1982). *Coercive Family Process.* Eugene, OR: Castalia.

Patterson, Gerald R., Patricia Chanberlain, and John B. Reid (1982). A comparative evaluation of a parent-training program. *Behavior Therapy* 13: 638-650.

Paulson, Morris J., Abdelmonem A. Afifi, Anne Chaleff, Vinnie Y. Liu, and Mary L. Thomason (1975). A discriminant function procedure for identifying abusive parents. *Suicide* 5: 104-114.

Polansky, Norman A., and James M. Gaudin (1983). Social distancing of the neglectful family. *Social Service Review* 57: 196-208.

Polansky, Norman A., P. Ammons, and James Gaudin (1985). Loneliness and isolation in child neglect. *Social Casework* 66: 338-347.

Polansky, Norman A., M.A. Chalmers, D.P. Williams, and E. William Buttenweiser (1981). *Damaged Parents: An Anatomy of Child Neglect.* Chicago, IL: University of Chicago Press.

Powell, John (1972). *Why Am I Afraid to Love?* Niles, IL: Argus Communications Co.

Remocker, Jane A., and Elizabeth T. Storch (1987). *Action Speaks Louder: A Handbook of Structured Group Techniques.* New York: Churchill Livingstone.

Shapiro, Deborah (1980). A CWLA study of factors involved in child abuse. *Child Welfare* 59: 242-243.

Sherrod, Kathryn B., William A. Altmeier, Susan O'Conner, and Peter M. Vietze (1984). Early prediction of child maltreatment. *Early Child Development and Care* 13: 335-350.

Stevens, John O. (1971). *Awareness: Explaining, Experimenting, Experiences.* Newark, CA: Real People Publishing.

Strauss, M.A. (1980). Social stress and marital violence in a national sample of American families. *Forensic Psychology and Psychiatry* 347: 229-250.

Timberlake, Elizabeth M., and Sandra S. Chipungu (1992). Grandmotherhood: Contemporary meaning among African-American middle-class grandmothers. *Social Work* 37: 216-222.

Wahler, Robert G., and Jean E. Dumas (1984). Changing the observational coding styles of insular and noninsular mothers: A step toward maintenance of parent-training effects. In Richard F. Dangel and Richard A. Polster (Eds.), *Parent Training: Foundations of Research and Practice.* New York: Guilford.

Weintraub, Marsha, and Barbara Wolf (1983). Effects of stress and social supports on mother-child interactions in single and two-parent families. *Child Development* 54: 1297-1311.

Whittaker, James K., and Elizabeth M. Tracy (1988). Social network intervention in intensive family-based preventive services. *Prevention in Human Services* 9: 175-192.

Young, Gay and Tamra Gately (1988). Neighborhood impoverishment and child maltreatment: An analysis from the ecological perspective. *Journal of Family Issues* 9 (2): 240-254.

Zuravin, Susan, and Geoffrey L. Greif (1989). Normative and child-maltreating AFDC mothers. *Social Casework* 70: 76-84.

Video References:

Hot Makeup, Tips for that Cool Look. Plymouth, MN: Simitar Entertainment, Inc.

Revelli, Clare (1987). *Color and You.* New York: Simon and Schuster Video.

Women's Health Issues. "Things My Mother Never Told Me," Perennial Education, Inc. Evanston, IL: Schul Group Corp.

Musical References:

Brooks, Garth. (1991) "The River," from the cassette, *Ropin' the Wind.* Nashville, TN: Capitol Nashville, a division of Capitol-EMI Music, Inc.

Recommended Readings for Parents

Baer, Jean (1976). *How to Be an Assertive (Not Aggressive) Woman in Life, in Love, and on the Job.* New York: Penguin Books USA, Inc.

Branden, Nathaniel (1983). *Honoring the Self.* New York: Bantam Books.

Burns, David, MD (1985). *Intimate Connections.* New York: Signet.

Capacchione, Lucia (1982). *The Creative Journal for Children.* Boston, MA: Shambhala.

Carpenter, Zerle L., Director Texas Agricultural Extension Service (1990). *Eating Right is Basic* and other publications. Austin, TX: Texas Agricultural Service.

Carter, Steve (1990). *What Smart Women Know.* New York: M. Evans.

Clarke, Jean Illsley (1978). *Self-Esteem: A Family Affair.* California: Harper & Row.

Cole-Whittaker, Terry (1989). *Love and Power in a World Without Limits.* New York: Harper & Row.

Drakeford, John W. (1976). *Do You Hear Me, Honey?* New York: Harper & Row.

Fluegelman, Andrew (1981). *More New Games.* Berkeley, CA: Headlands Press.

Forward, Dr. Susan (1989). *Toxic Parents.* New York: Bantam Books.

Hendricks, Gay, PhD (1990). *Learning to Love Yourself Workbook.* New York: Prentice Hall.

John-Roger and Peter McWilliams (1991). *Life 101.* Los Angeles, CA: Prelude Press.

Johnson, Barbara (1990). *Pain Is Inevitable but Misery Is Optional.* Dallas, TX: Word Publishing.

Johnson, Barbara (1992). *Splashes of Joy in the Cesspools of Life.* Dallas, TX: Word Publishing.

Johnson, Barbara (1993). *Pack Up Your Gloomees in a Great Big Box, Then Sit on the Lid and Laugh!* Dallas, TX: Word Publishing.

Kagan, Richard and Shirley Schlosberg (1989). *Families in Perpetual Crisis.* New York: W. W. Norton and Company, Inc.

Leman, Kevin (1987). *The Pleasers, Women Who Can't Say NO—and the Men Who Control Them.* New York: Dell Publishing.

Lennox, Joan Hatch and Judith Hatch Shapiro (1990). *Lifechanges.* New York: Crown Publishers, Inc.

Marone, Nicky (1992). *Women and Risk.* New York: St. Martin's Press.

Matthews, Andrew (1988). *Being Happy.* California: Price Stern Sloan, Inc.

Matthews, Andrew (1991). *Making Friends.* California: Price Stern Sloan, Inc.

McKay, Matthew, PhD, and Patrick Fanning (1987). *Self-Esteem.* Oakland, CA: Harbinger.

Miller, Keith, and Andrea Wells Miller (1981). *The Single Experience.* Dallas, TX: Word Publishing.

Palmer, Pat, EdD (1977). *Liking Myself.* San Luis Obispo, CA: Impact Publishers.

Paul, Jordan, PhD, and Margaret Paul, PhD (1987). *If You Really Loved Me.* Minneapolis, MN: CompCare Publishers.

Phelps, Stanlee, and Nancy Austin (1985). *The Assertive Woman.* San Luis Obispo, CA: Impact Publishers.

Pilkington, Maya, and the Diagram Group (1987). *The Real Life Aptitude Test.* New York: Pharos Books.

Semigran, Candace (1988). *One Minute Self Esteem—Caring for Yourself and Others.* New York: Bantam Books.

Sheperd, Scott, PhD (1990). *What Do You Think of YOU?* Minneapolis, MN: CompCare Publishers.

Sherman, Robert, and Norman Fredman (1986). *Handbook of Structured Techniques in Marriage and Family Therapy.* New York: Brunner/Mazel, Inc.

Texas Department of Human Services. *Assertiveness for Neglecting Mothers.* Austin, TX: TDHS.

Thoele, Sue Patton (1988). *The Courage to Be Yourself.* Nevada City, CA: Pyramid Press.

Viscott, David (1977). *Risking.* New York: Simon and Schuster.

Woititz, Janet G., EdD (1992). *Healthy Parenting.* New York: Simon and Schuster/Fireside.

Index

Page numbers followed by the letter "t" indicate a table.

Reid, John B., 4
Relationships (week three), 61-63
Relaxation exercise, 156-157
Remocker, Jane A., 63,88,162
Research, supporting LAMS, 2-5
Results (Learning About Myself),
    171,173,175,178,179,
    181-182
Revelli, Clare, 83
Richey, Cheryl A., 4,168
Rickard, Verna, 6
Risk and strengths assessment, 168
"River, The," 152,155
Role-play, 51,52,57-58,117
  put downs, 123-124
  What Do You Do?, 76-77
Ropin' the Wind (Garth Brooks),
    152,155
Running LAMS, 15-20

Sample (Learning About Myself),
    170
Seasonal special, 132
Self (week one), 33-36
Self-esteem. *See also* IALAC;
    Poison statements
  low, 2
Self-talk, 55
Shapiro, Deborah, 2,16,168
Sherrod, Kathryn B., 2
Shopping. *See* Financial
    responsibility
Smart shopping, 130-132
Smell-A-Spice (game), 144
Social isolation, 181
Social networks, enhancements
    to, 181
"Spaghetti Structures," 161,164
Speaker
  on health, 113-114
  on homemaking skills, 138
  on nutrition, 148

"Spears and Cheers," 116,118-119
Spice List, 144-145
Staples, 131
Storch, Elizabeth T., 63,88,162
Strauss, M.A., 168
Support system, LAMS as, 10

Temper. *See* Anger
Texas Department of Protective
    and Regulatory Services, 171
Theme, 18
Things My Mother Never Told Me,
    114
"This is My Nose," 154
Timberlake, Elizabeth M., 169
Time for oneself (week five), 85-88
Tracy, Elizabeth M., 168
Transportation, problem with, 8

"Ungame," 95,101

Wahler, Robert G., 3
Weekly evaluation, 25
Weintraub, Marsha, 2-3
Wells, Harold, 52,108,119,128
"What Things Can I Do Well?,"
    104,108-109
Whelan, J.P., 168
When I (game), 34,37-39
Whittaker, James K., 168
Why Am I Afraid to Love?, 56
Wolf, Barbara, 3

"You" statements, 70
Young, Gay, 2,3,6
"You've Got It - I Want It," 52,54

Zuravin, Susan, 168

Order Your Own Copy of
This Important Book for Your Personal Library!

THE LEARNING ABOUT MYSELF (LAMS) PROGRAM FOR AT-RISK PARENTS
Learning from the Past—Changing the Future

_____ in hardbound at $39.95 (ISBN: 0-7890-0107-1)

_____ in softbound at $24.95 (ISBN: 0-7890-0474-7)

COST OF BOOKS_____

OUTSIDE USA/CANADA/
MEXICO: ADD 20%_____

POSTAGE & HANDLING_____
*(US: $3.00 for first book & $1.25
for each additional book)
Outside US: $4.75 for first book
& $1.75 for each additional book)*

SUBTOTAL_____

IN CANADA: ADD 7% GST_____

STATE TAX_____
*(NY, OH & MN residents, please
add appropriate local sales tax)*

FINAL TOTAL_____
*(If paying in Canadian funds,
convert using the current
exchange rate. UNESCO
coupons welcome.)*

☐ **BILL ME LATER:** ($5 service charge will be added)
(Bill-me option is good on US/Canada/Mexico orders only;
not good to jobbers, wholesalers, or subscription agencies.)

☐ Check here if billing address is different from
shipping address and attach purchase order and
billing address information.

Signature_____

☐ **PAYMENT ENCLOSED: $**_____

☐ **PLEASE CHARGE TO MY CREDIT CARD.**

☐ Visa   ☐ MasterCard   ☐ AmEx   ☐ Discover

Account # _____

Exp. Date _____

Signature _____

Prices in US dollars and subject to change without notice.

NAME _____

INSTITUTION _____

ADDRESS _____

CITY _____

STATE/ZIP _____

COUNTRY _____ COUNTY (NY residents only) _____

TEL _____ FAX _____

E-MAIL_____
May we use your e-mail address for confirmations and other types of information? ☐ Yes   ☐ No

Order From Your Local Bookstore or Directly From
The Haworth Press, Inc.
10 Alice Street, Binghamton, New York 13904-1580 • USA
TELEPHONE: 1-800-HAWORTH (1-800-429-6784) / Outside US/Canada: (607) 722-5857
FAX: 1-800-895-0582 / Outside US/Canada: (607) 772-6362
E-mail: getinfo@haworth.com
PLEASE PHOTOCOPY THIS FORM FOR YOUR PERSONAL USE.

BOF96